Trace Elements in Health and Disease

Trace Elements in Health and Disease

Edited by

Antero Aitio
Institute of Occupational Health, Finland
Antti Aro
National Public Health Institute, Finland
Jorma Järvisalo
Social Insurance Institution, Finland
Harri Vainio
International Agency for Research on Cancer, France

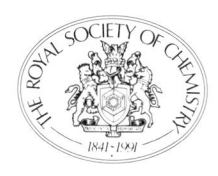

British Library Cataloguing in Publication Data
Joint Nordic Elements Society/ Commission on Toxicology
 International Symposium (*1990. Espoo, Finland*)
 Trace elements in health and disease.
 1. Man. Trace elements
 I. Title II. Aitio, Antero III. Royal Society of Chemistry
 612.3924

ISBN 0-85186-976-9

Proceedings of a joint Nordic Trace Element Society/Union of Pure and Applied Chemistry International Symposium on Trace Elements in Health and Disease held 5-8 June 1990 in Espoo, Finland

© The Royal Society of Chemistry 1991

All Rights Reserved
No part of this book may be reproduced or transmitted in any form
or by any means — graphic, electronic, including photocopying,
recording, taping or information storage and retrieval systems —
without written permission from The Royal Society of Chemistry

Published by The Royal Society of Chemistry,
Thomas Graham House, Science Park, Cambridge
CB4 4WF

Printed and bound in Great Britain by
Bookcraft (Bath) Ltd.

Preface

During the last decade trace elements have been the target of intensive research. This interest has focused on the different aspects of toxicity, mechanisms thereof, and on the role of trace elements in nutrition, especially their essentiality in the diet of humans. Although some elements have been studied for both these aspects —essentiality and long-term toxic effects (eg of nickel, chromium, and cobalt)— research in these two areas has been separated. The purpose of the International Symposium on Trace Elements in Health and Disease, held on 5-8 June 1990 in Espoo, Finland, was to gather together those who are interested in analytical, metabolic, nutritional or toxicological aspects of trace element research, with the purpose of reviewing the current state of knowledge on the relationship between trace elements and human health and disease. Special attention was given also to trace elements and other micronutrients with antioxidant properties. This volume is a compilation of the major contributions made in the Symposium.

The Symposium was a joint meeting under the auspices of the Nordic Trace Element Society (NTES) - and the Commission on Toxicology of the Clinical Chemistry Division of the International Union of Pure and Applied Chemistry (IUPAC), and followed the traditions of the NTES and COMTOX meetings that previously have been organized separately. The Symposium was organized by the Finnish Institute of Occupational Health, the National Public Health Institute and the Social Insurance Institution, Finland. Financial support from the Finnish Work Environment Fund, and the Ministry of Education, Finland is gratefully acknowledged.

The editors.

Contents

Analytical Methods and Quality Control

Advances in the Detection of Trace Elements in Biological Fluids and Tissues
J. Savory and M. R. Wills — 3

Principal Components Analysis for the Determination of Ni in Urine by ICP-MS
Douglas M. Templeton and Margaret-Anne Vaughan — 19

Atomic Fluorescence Spectrometry for the Determination of Mercury in Biological Samples
G. Vermeir, C. Vandecasteele, and R. Dams — 29

Quality Assurance : Achievements, Problems, Prospects
S. S. Brown — 37

Exposure and Exposure Assessment

Selenium in Tap Water and Natural Water Ecosystems in Finland
Dacheng Wang, Georg Alfthan, Antti Aro, Lea Kauppi, and Jouko Soveri — 49

Release of Aluminium from Coated Saucepans
Andrew Taylor — 57

Constraints in Biological Monitoring
Philippe Grandjean — 65

Heavy Metals in the General Population: Trend Evaluation and Interrelation with Trace Elements
B. Heinzow, H. Jessen, S. Mohr, and D. Riemer — 75

Trace Element Levels in the Hair, Blood, Cord Blood and Placenta of Pregnant Women from Central Slovenia
M. Horvat, A. Prosenc, J. Smrke, D. Konda, A.R. Byrne, P. Stegnar, and I. Begic — 83

Kinetics of Heavy Metals

Cadmium Toxicokinetics Following Long-term
Occupational Exposure
R.A. Braithwaite, R. Armstrong,
D.M. Franklin, D.R. Chettle, and M.C. Scott
   95

Absorption of Bismuth from Two Bismuth Salts
during *in Vivo* Perfusion of the Rat Small
Intestine
A. Slikkerveer, G.B. van der Voet, and
F.A. de Wolff
   105

Transfer of Lead via Rat Milk and Tissue Uptake
in the Suckling Offspring
I. Palminger and A. Oskarsson
   109

Milk Transfer of Mercury in Rats Given Inorganic
or Methylmercury
J. Sundberg and A. Oskarsson
   117

Micronutrients in Human Health

Micronutrients and Cardiovascular Disease
J. Virtamo and J.K. Huttunen
   127

The Epidemiology of Selenium and Human Cancer
W. C. Willett, M. J. Stampfer, D. Hunter, and
G. A. Colditz
   141

Carcinogenicity and Teratogenicity of Metals

On the Carcinogenicity of Nickel and Chromium
and Their Compounds
A. Aitio and L. Tomatis
   159

Teratogenicity of Ni^{2+} in *Xenopus Laevis*
S.M. Hopfer, M.C. Plowman, K.R. Sweeney,
J.A. Bantle, and F.W. Sunderman, Jr.
   169

Mechanisms of Action of Trace Elements

The Significance of Target Cells for a Model of
Uptake and Biological Transformation of αNi_3S_2
H.F. Hildebrand, P. Shirali, F.Z. Arrouijal,
A.M. Decaestecker, and R. Martinez
   179

Oxygen Free Radicals, Other Reactive Species and
Antioxidants
J. O. Järvisalo
   191

Free Radicals, Lipid Peroxidation   201
  and Human Disease
  T.L.Dormandy

Metal-Proteoglycan Interactions in the   209
  Regulation of Renal Mesangial Cells:
  Implications for Metal-Induced Nephropathy
  Douglas M. Templeton

Application of an Organ Culture Matrix System   219
  to Neurotoxicity Studies in the Foetal Rabbit
  Midbrain
  *C. D. Hewitt, M. M. Herman, J. Savory, and
  M. R. Wills*

Effects of Aluminium Maltol on Brain Tissue   227
  in Vivo and *in Vitro*
  *M. R. Wills, C. D. Hewitt, J. Savory, and
  M. M. Herman*

Analytical Methods and Quality Control

Advances in the Detection of Trace Elements in Biological Fluids and Tissues

J. Savory and M. R. Wills

DEPTS. OF PATHOLOGY, INTERNAL MEDICINE AND BIOCHEMISTRY, UNIVERSITY OF VIRGINIA HEALTH SCIENCES CENTER, CHARLOTTESVILLE, VIRGINIA 22908, USA

1 INTRODUCTION

In the 13 years since the first International Symposium on the Clinical Chemistry and Chemical Toxicology of Metals held at Monte Carlo 25 March 1977, considerable advances have been made in our knowledge of this subject. As we unravel the basic mechanisms of action of essential and toxic metals new tools of biomedical science are being applied. Foremost in recent years are the techniques of molecular biology and use of immunoprobes particularly monoclonal antibodies. High resolution separation techniques also have numerous applications, particularly high performance liquid chromatography. However, the direct measurement of the metal itself in biological fluid or tissue still remains of importance in studying both metal toxicity and nutritional deficiencies. Clinical diagnosis, monitoring in the clinic or workplace, or research, all require guidelines for specimen collection, contamination control, and accurate, precise and sensitive analytical techniques. For clinical and occupational monitoring, bulk analysis of fluid or tissue is the most practical assay. However, frequently there is a need in the research laboratory to localize trace amounts of metals in tissues. In addition, the achievement and maintenance of high quality analytical results requires the availability of standard reference materials and proficiency test specimens. Target values for such materials can be achieved by a consensus of results which may be in error, or by the application of definitive analytical methods. The present review covers some advances in analytical techniques over the past few years.

The older chemical and physicochemical methods once used extensively for metal measurements in biological materials has been replaced with newer techniques of which atomic spectroscopy especially atomic absorption has become the most widely used. For more definitive analyses mass spectrometric techniques have provided enhanced accuracy.

2 ATOMIC ABSORPTION SPECTROMETRY

General Considerations

For some of the more common clinical chemistry measurements such as calcium, magnesium, zinc and copper, flame atomization techniques perform well. Such methods are relatively simple in this mode of operation, have modest cost and possess moderately sensitive limits of detection.

Electrothermal atomization continues to be the workhorse for the more challenging trace metal analyses. In a review by Slavin[1] electrochemical atomic absorption spectrometry (EAAS) is stated to be the most sensitive spectroscopic technique having detection limits 10 to 100 times better than flame atomic absorption or inductively coupled plasma (ICP) emission. Sensitivity is often 1000 times better on an absolute mass basis. Serious limitations of EAAS particularly for the analysis of biological specimens have been the interferences. Although EAAS is not completely interference-free, there have been vast improvements by using high-quality graphite combined with platform technology. Carbon-based materials are by far the most widely used for the manufacture of electrothermal atomizers. A combination of pyrolytically coated tubes and either pyrolytic graphite or glassy carbon platforms are recommended for optimal EAAS performance.[1,2] Such performance is also achieved by new instrument developments with more reproducible temperature control, fast photometric instrumentation and Zeeman background correction allowing ultratrace analyses in the sub parts per billion range to be performed.

Matrix Modification

The use of matrix modifiers has contributed immensely in reducing interferences in EAAS analyses. The chemical reactions involved in the stabilization of specific elements by a matrix modifier are interesting, complex and mostly one has to deal with each specific analyte at a time. Nickel nitrate has been used extensively as a matrix modifier[3-5] but cannot be recommended for hospital laboratories where nickel analyses are part of the test repertoire. Palladium is being used frequently as a replacement for nickel.[6-9] For selenium measurements it provides a much cleaner signal ie., less background and, thus, enhances the sensitivity. Palladium as a matrix modifier does have applications for several elements. The combination of palladium with magnesium nitrate has been suggested as a general purpose matrix modifier.[10] To illustrate the point that each individual element has its own requirements for matrix modification, we present a selection of modifiers used in our own laboratory. Aluminium when measured using the stabilized temperature platform requires magnesium nitrate whereas aluminium analysis without the platform requires nitric acid. Arsenic and selenium use palladium chloride, cadmium, copper and lead require ammonium hydrogen phosphate, manganese employs nitric acid plus magnesium nitrate, chromium and nickel employ an initial precipitation step with nitric acid and thus have hydrogen ion in the final mixture, and zinc requires no matrix modifier. An understanding of the chemical reactions between the analyte, matrix modifier and furnace material has been the subject of many investigations [9,11] and such information undoubtedly leads to the optimal use of modifiers.

A disadvantage of EAAS is that it is a slow technique taking several minutes per sample analysed, and the use of the stabilized temperature platform often increases the analysis time appreciably. In the authors' laboratory aluminium measurements in plasma are performed by one of two methods depending on the clinical requirements.[12] For subjects with normal renal function where the serum aluminium is usually less than 0.370 µmol/L we use magnesium nitrate as the matrix modifier[13-16] with concomitant use of a stabilized temperature platform and an oxygen-ash step at 600°C. Using this method the lowest concentration of aluminium detectable is 0.037 µmol/L with a characteristic mass of 16.3 pg/0.0044 A.s and a detection limit of 10 pg. Using this method only seven samples per hour can be analysed. There are considerable differences between plasma aluminium concentrations in healthy subjects and patients with impaired renal function. In the latter category serum aluminium may be increased 100-fold over normal; in addition also many more requests are made of the clinical chemistry laboratory since aluminium monitoring is carried out 3-4 times per year in all patients on hemodialysis treatment. In these patients excellent precision is required but sensitivity is not of prime importance. For these analyses we dispense with the use of the stabilized temperature platform and employ 0.1 mmol/L nitric acid as a matrix modifier as reported previously.[17] The lowest concentration of aluminium detectable in a sample using this method is 0.133 µmol/L with a characteristic mass of 26.6 pg/0.0044 A.s and a detection limit of 16 pg. This sensitivity is adequate for the specimens being analysed and the throughput is seventeen samples per hour. In contrast to the first method we estimate the second method to be half as expensive.

Absolute Analysis

Theoretically it is now possible to perform absolute analysis with EAAS since there are a number of characteristics unique to these techniques. L'vov et al[18] using integrated absorbance signals compared calculated values for the characteristic mass with those obtained experimentally for forty elements. For thirty of the elements the calculated characteristic mass averaged ninety percent of that determined experimentally. It has been stated by other workers[19] that the longitudinal temperature gradient in the furnace is the limiting factor for absolute analysis.

Hydride Generation Techniques

Hydride generation techniques continue to be applied effectively as a means of volatilizing some metals. These techniques provide a means of isolating the element from the sample matrix as well as providing some degree of concentration. Thus, sensitivity is improved and spectral interferences are reduced. Elements which lend themselves to hydride generation techniques are antimony, arsenic, bismuth, germanium, selenium and tin. However, care is needed since hydride generation techniques are subject to interferences arising from hydride production and transport processes.[20] Boampong et al[21] have demonstrated such an interference by L-cystine in the hydride generation method for arsenic. These authors also review briefly the subject of interferences in hydride generation techniques especially in the determination of arsenic. Several elements reduce the signal from arsenic; cobalt(II), nickel(II), palladium(II), and platinum(IV) having marked effects.[22]

Multielement Analysis

Simultaneous multielement detection can be achieved by a combination of continuous source atomic absorption spectrometry with electrothermal atomization. This type of system has several advantages including simple optical configurations, background correction and low detection limits provided the wavelength is above 250 nm. These techniques have poor source intensity below 250 nm. Jones et al[23] report a system using photodiode array detection and provide a means of observing and correcting for broad band background absorption and spectral interferences, directly in the acquired spectrum without the need for wavelength modulation. Parameters and detection limits for nineteen elements were reported,[23] the latter ranging for 0.1 pg for magnesium to 700 pg for arsenic.

3 INDUCTIVELY COUPLED PLASMA EMISSION (ICP)

This technique will not be reviewed in detail in the present paper. However, ICP has many advantages over other techniques in that it has multielement capabilities, does not require a special source for each element, has a wide concentration range, and lends itself to automation. On the whole, detection limits of ICP compare favorably with flame atomic absorption spectrometry and interferences generally are fewer.

4 LASER FLUORESCENCE AND LASER IONIZATION

The more conventional analytical techniques described above will allow the measurement of trace metals in the low parts per billion range provided the specimen is not diluted appreciably prior to analysis. Inductively coupled plasma-mass spectrometry (ICP-MS) has similar detection limits to EAAS, being slightly more sensitive in some instances. Laser fluorescence and laser ionization approaches possess a detection power of parts per quadrillion concentration. The response for these incredible sensitivity limits which approach single atom detection is because, unlike all other methods, they are not limited either by instrumental and system noise, and by detection efficiencies much less than unity. For example the detection efficiency of atomic absorption is much lower than unity since a light beam can never be focused to a diameter equal to the absorption cross section. Mass spectrometric detection has an overall efficiency no better than 10^{-5} in the atomization-ionization-interfacing. Laser fluorescence and laser ionization techniques approach the ideal. The efficiency of detection must be unity in order to achieve single atom detection i.e. every atom produced for the sample must produce a detectable event. Another important factor is that instrumental and atomizer noises must be less than the intrinsic noises. Absolute experimental detection limits for laser excited atomic fluorescence spectrometry (LEAFS) is 0.5-5 fg, laser enhanced ionization (LEI) 5-50 fg which can be compared to EAAS 0.2-100 pg and ICP-MS > 50 pg. Whether these approaches will be used for routine analyses of complex samples is still debatable. However, they have incredible potential for the research worker interested in metal toxicology.

5 MASS SPECTROMETRY

Isotope specific analytical methods or isotope dilution mass spectrometry (IDMS) can be contrasted with element-specific methods used in classical analytical chemistry. Isotope-specific methods can provide the most accurate measurements of elemental concentrations because of their high degree of specificity. Most often thermal ionization mass spectrometers designed specifically for isotope ratio measurements have been used for these analyses.[24-28] Such instruments are so specialized that they are not readily available to the toxicologist; rather their applications are in the nuclear industry. Two other techniques, ICP-MS and applications of organic mass spectrometers are presented here.

Inductively Coupled Plasma - Mass Spectrometry

Gray[29] was the first to describe the mass spectrometric elemental analysis of ions extracted from a high temperature dc plasma. This work led to the development of ICP-MS.[30,31] The main feature of this technique is its capability of providing both elemental and isotopic measurements with a high degree of sensitivity, wide dynamic range and multielement analysis capabilities. An ICP which is a well-established ion source in emission spectroscopy, is interfaced with a quadrupole mass spectrometer. The technical difficulties of such an interface are obvious when one component is a plasma of gas (5000°K) at atmospheric pressure, and the other a high vacuum mass spectrometer. The technique has been shown using NBS-SRM bovine liver to provide accurate results for aluminium, barium, chromium, copper, iron, manganese, molybdenum, nickel and zinc.[32] In the same study appreciable polyatomic interferences were observed when the analysis of urine was attempted indicating that an initial chemical separation step would be necessary.

One major feature of elemental analysis by mass spectrometry is its potential for performing animal and human clinical studies of elemental bioavailability by using stable isotopes. For example zinc bioavailability has been studied by plasma analysis after oral ingestion of ^{70}Zn.[33]

Now with the availability of commercial ICP-MS instruments, this technique has immense potential to routine analysis and to research in the field of trace metals.

Organic Mass Spectrometry

The potential of general purpose mass spectrometers for trace metal determinations has been demonstrated in a few publications. Gas chromatography-mass spectrometry (GC-MS) has been successfully used for isotope ratio measurements for two metals: chromium in biological materials[34] and sea water[35] and selenium in biological materials.[36] The lack of suitable chelating agents has been one of the limitations preventing the wider application of GC-MS. Problems with the use of metal chelates have been the poor accuracy of the isotope ratio measurements[37-39] and exchange of the metal in the chelate with the metals in the GC-MS system, causing cross-contamination during sequential analyses of samples of widely varying isotopic compositions.[40-42] Some of the studies reported, therefore, have not measured isotope ratios but rather have depended on the use of integrated ion currents for quantitation.[41,43]

We have developed a GC-MS method involving thermally stable, volatile chelates. We investigated measurement of isotope ratios of chromium, nickel, zinc and copper.[44] The chelating agents acetylacetone, trifluoroacetylacetone, sodium diethyldithiocarbamate and lithium bis(trifluoroethyl)dithiocarbamate were used. Experimental conditions for the preparation of chelates and the mass spectrometric operating parameters for precise and accurate measurement of isotope ratios were optimized using a general-purpose mass spectrometer. Imprecision values of 1-4% were obtained for measurements of different isotope ratios using chelates containing about 10 ng of metal. The capability of this technique for the accurate determination of natural and altered isotope ratios was also evaluated for these elements using lithium bis(trifluoroethyl)dithiocarbamate as a chelating agent. This GC-MS method obviates the need for a more specialized mass spectrometer such as a thermal ionization or inductively coupled plasma mass spectrometer for trace metal determinations.

We further applied this technique to the measurement of nickel[45] in serum and urine and chromium[46] in urine. Both methods again use lithium bis(trifluoroethyl)dithiocarbamate as a chelating agent with subsequent isotope ratios being monitored following capillary column GC-MS analysis. The memory effect between samples of different isotope ratios was evaluated and found to be negligible. The accuracy of each method was verified by the analysis of National Institute of Standards and Technology (NIST) freeze-dried urine reference material SRM-2670, for which acceptable results were obtained.

A key feature of these GC-MS procedures is that they use conventional instruments available now in many laboratories engaged in drug testing. However, sample preparation is tedious and prone to contamination. Also, sensitivity is not quite as good as EAAS. It seems probable that ICP-MS will be more widely used. However, for some specific applications GC-MS will fulfill certain needs.

6 ROBOTICS

Trace metal analysis is complicated considerably by contamination. We discuss this problem later both in respect to reagent contamination and the need to work in a clean environment. In the future one means by which contamination will be controlled during specimen handling, will be by the use of robotics. Metal contamination from a human operator will be minimized. Robotics offers a excellent means of providing high quality analyses, increased throughput and reduced costs. Systems need to be designed with built in checks for integrity of analysis in order to ensure that errors will be recognized. At the present time few, if any, laboratories are using robotics for trace metal measurements. However, as more laboratories become familiar with the potential of robotics, then the applications will be developed. The authors, have been engaged in robotic development in clinical chemistry[47] and foresee wide applications.

7 MICROANALYSIS

All of the analytical techniques discussed previously in this review have been for bulk analysis of biological specimens. In order to obtain distinct localization of elements within tissues, it is necessary to combine microscopy with analytical techniques. Using microanalysis a correlation is obtained between the structure of a microscopic cellular component and its chemical composition.

Microanalysis in the transmission electron microscope is most commonly performed using the energy-dispersive x-ray spectroscopy technique. This method has been used for many years and many procedures for specimen preparation and analysis have been developed and refined. More recently a transmission electron microscope with an incorporated electron spectrometer has become available commercially which now allows the use of electron energy loss spectroscopy (EELS) in biomedical research. Electron beam instruments are not the only means of providing elemental microanalysis. The laser microprobe uses irradiation with a laser beam to ionize a specific part of the specimen, followed by analysis of the ions generated in a time of flight mass spectrometer. The ion microprobe uses the secondary ions from the specimen generated by bombardment with a primary ion beam. The proton microprobe uses the x-ray spectrum generated by a beam of high energy protons. As is evident from this brief introduction, all microanalytical techniques are different in principle, instrumentation and performance such as sensitivity and spatial resolution.

Examples of applications of some of these techniques is given for the authors' main area of interest which is aluminium toxicity.

Energy-dispersive X-ray Analysis (EDS)

Energy-dispersive x-ray analysis has been used to localize aluminium deposits within the glomerular basement membrane.[48] Using this same technique Perl et al[49] examined brain tissue from patients with amyotrophic lateral sclerosis and parkinsonism-dementia, and located aluminium in neurofibrillary tangle-bearing hippocampal neurons. Other workers also using this technique have localized aluminium in bone tissues.[50,51] In experimental animals the technique has been used for the ultrastructural localization of aluminium in brains for rats given aluminium chloride injections.[52]

Laser Microprobe Mass Analysis (LAMMA)

The Laser Microprobe Mass Analyser provides high lateral resolution and extreme detection sensitivity. The instrument consists of a pulsed Nd-YAG laser (265 nm), an optical microscope, a time-of-flight mass spectrometer with an open secondary electron multiplier and suitable detection electronics. The principle of LAMMA is based on the excitation of a microvolume of the sample to an ionized state by a focused laser beam. The analytical information is derived from mass spectrometry of these ions. This technique has been used to localize aluminium in the lysosomes of hepatocytes as well as Kupffer cells from liver tissue of patients on chronic hemodialysis.[53,54] We recently have used LAMMA to study the ultrastructural localization of aluminium in livers of aluminium maltol-treated rabbits.[55]

Electron Energy Loss Spectroscopy (EELS)

A technique complementary to x-ray microanalysis is EELS, where the information carried by the electrons that have originally caused the x-ray excitation in the specimen, is studied. In this technique, electrons that have passed through the specimen are separated according to their kinetic energy by an electron spectrometer to form a high resolution energy spectrum. The electron energy loss spectrum, which represents the graphical display of the energy lost by the electrons scattered by the specimen versus the corresponding electron intensity, can be analysed directly, or a signal from a specifically chosen part of the spectrum can be passed on to form an image. This technique provides exceptionally good resolution even though the original promise of excellent sensitivity has not materialized. The principles of the technique are given in two excellent reviews.[56,57] We have applied this technique to the analysis of liver from aluminium maltol-treated rabbits.[58]

A major problem with microanalysis of tissue is in the processing of the specimen. Conventional chemical fixation as developed for morphological studies, is not ideal for localizing trace elements. Movement of metal ions within the cell must be a serious consideration as tissues are left for several days in a fixative. We presently use rapid freezing and freeze substitution as a means of tissue processing, but these techniques are extremely difficult.

Although both the LAMMA and EELS require very expensive sophisticated equipment, both are extremely powerful techniques for studying metal localization in tissues. The sensitivity of the LAMMA technique appears to be better than EELS but the resolution of the latter techniques is better. Our understanding of the toxicity of metals will be aided considerably by the use of such localization techniques.

8   SPECIMEN HANDLING

Specimen Collection

Many different types of specimens are submitted for trace element measurements. The most common are biological fluids usually serum (or plasma) and urine, although there is sometimes interest in cerebrospinal fluid. Tissue analysis is also of importance and the laboratory must be equipped to analyse a wide variety of tissues such as bone, brain, muscle, liver, etc. Hair analysis has gained some interest but it should be discouraged in most instances since contamination from the environment and shampoos is a major problem. Recently, because of the high level of interest in aluminium toxicity in hemodialysis patients, dialysis water and dialysate solutions are commonly analysed. General aspects of specimen collection, processing and storage have been reviewed by Aitio and Järvisalo[59] and also by Seiler.[60]

The present authors recommend for trace metal measurements such as aluminium, copper and zinc that an acid-washed plastic syringe be used with a stainless steel needle, and that the blood be transferred to a polypropylene tube (Falcon, Oxnard CA) for processing and storage. An alternate approach which is satisfactory for aluminium is to use a plastic collection tube containing uncontaminated lithium heparinate as an anticoagulant. Even greater care must be taken for ultra trace analysis such as the measurement of chromium, cobalt or nickel in serum. The blood collection technique must not allow the specimen to come into contact with a metal needle, and to circumvent this problem we collect our specimen into an acid-washed polypropylene test tube using a needle with a teflon or polyethylene intravenous catheter.[61]

Procedures for the collection and storage of urine and faecal specimens have been developed in our laboratory.[62] Twenty-four hour urine specimens are collected in plastic containers (Scientific Products, McGraw Park, IL) and an aliquot transferred and stored at 4°C in a polypropylene tube (Falcon, Oxnard, CA). Faecal specimens are collected directly into plastic bags, weighed and frozen.

Sources of Contamination in Analysis

Every item used during analysis is a possible source of trace metal contamination. To be considered are such items as glass- and plasticware, pipette tips, collection tubes, sample cups, purity of reagents, standards, acids, water and the working environment. Contamination of glass- and plasticware is removed by acid washing and all acids should be ultrapure grade. Techniques for preparing exceptionally high purity acids have been reported.[63-65] Water should produce a resistivity of at least 18 megohms and continuous monitoring is necessary. The room chosen for analysis should have limited access to ensure a clean working environment and powder-free gloves must be worn at all times. Sample preparation should be carried out in an environmental laminar flow hood. We use a filter unit (122 x 61 cm) suspended from the ceiling with plastic sheeting enclosed to bench level. This filter unit (MAC 10, Envirco, Hagerstown, MD) is inexpensive, convenient and provides class 100 air. Several units can be used together to provide more bench space having a clean air environment.

Sample Preparation for Analysis

A wide variety of sample preparation methods have been used, the level of complexity being dependent on the final analytical technique used.

For EAAS of biological fluids we use the following four procedures depending on the analyte: (i) dilution and direct analysis with external calibration, (ii) direct analysis with standard additions, (iii) digestion and extraction and (iv) protein precipitation.

The first of these procedures is the most straightforward and should be used whenever possible. Ideally the standard curve is constructed using aqueous standards. However if the sample matrix causes problems then matrix based calibrators may be used. Some workers[15] have used this approach for serum aluminium by preparing standards in a serum pool containing a minimal amount of endogenous aluminium. Standard additions can be used to minimize matrix effects but this approach inherently is imprecise since multiple analytical measurements, each with its own imprecisions, are made to achieve the final result. A valuable technique for the determination of nickel, and aluminium in serum is to precipitate proteins using a small amount of ultrapure concentrated nitric acid.[66,67] The final preparation which is relatively protein free has markedly reduced matrix effects.

Urine samples similarly may be simply diluted prior to EAAS measurement,[15] although acid digestion is often necessary. Analysis of faeces is more complicated and the procedure we use is as follows.[68] Frozen specimens are thawed and weighed in the original plastic container used for collection. Deionized water is added (1 ml per 2 g faeces) and the sample is homogenized on a paint shaker in a sealed paint can. A 10-ml aliquot is ashed, dissolved in dilute HNO_3, and analysed by EAAS.

Soft tissue samples, such as brain, liver, or muscle, must be homogenized before processing, and this can be accomplished easily by pummelling the tissue in a "Stomacher" blender (Fisher Scientific Company, Pittsburgh, PA 15219). Deionized water (5 ml) is added to the bag with the tissue. The sealed bag is placed in the blender and blended for 5-15 min, which completely homogenizes the sample. The homogenate can then be processed for analysis.

Microwave digestion of tissue specimens is a new technique which provides an excellent means of preparing a sample for EAAS without risking excessive contamination.[69] We use a microwave digestion bomb (Parr Instrument Company, Moline, IL 61265) which is modified with a teflon liner with a smaller sample well than the standard liner. Approximately 50 mg (100 mg maximum) of dried tissue plus 1 ml of 50% nitric acid are added to the teflon well. The bomb is sealed and placed in a standard microwave oven for approximately 1 minute. Elevated temperature and pressure promote rapid digestion of the tissue, while the sealed teflon liner eliminates external contamination and loss due to volatilization. Upon cooling the digest is ready for EAAS analysis.

9 CONCLUSIONS

Many advances have been made over the past decade in the detection of trace elements in biological fluids and tissues. As limits of detection are lowered then contamination problems increase dramatically. Almost certainly those methods requiring minimal sample preparation prior to analysis will be the ones most widely used. For this reason atomic spectroscopic methods will continue to be used extensively. Microprobe analysis for the trace metals still poses immense technical problems not least of which is tissue preparation. Very few investigators have access to the facilities to perform microprobe analyses, and yet application of these techniques are crucial to our understanding of mechanisms of action of essential and toxic metals.

Overall, the trace metal analyst is still presented with considerable challenges and important advances are achieved as these analytical hurdles are overcome.

10 REFERENCES

1. W. Slavin, *Anal. Chem.*, 1986, 58, 589A.
2. H. Guenther and B. Findeisen, *Freiberg. Forschungsh. A*, 1986, 730, 130.
3. A. Cedergren, I. Lindberg, E. Lundberg, D. C. Baxter and W. Frech, *Anal. Chim. Acta*, 1986, 180, 373.
4. J. Dedina, W. Frech, A. Cedergren, I. Lindburg and E. Lundberg, *J. Anal. At. Spectrom.*, 1987, 2, 435.
5. R. D. Ediger, *At. Absorpt. Newsl.*, 1975, 14, 127.
6. S. Xiao-quan, N. Zhe-ming and Z. Li, *At. Spectrosc.*, 1984, 5, 1.
7. S. Xiao-quan, N. Zhe-ming and Z. Li, *Talanta*, 1984, 31, 150.
8. S. Xiao-quan and H. Kaijin, *Talanta*, 1985, 32, 23.
9. S. Xiao-quan and W. Dian-Xun, *Anal. Chim. Acta*, 1985, 173, 315.
10. G. Schlemmer and B. Welz, *Spectrochim. Acta*, 1986, 41B, 1157.
11. B. S. Lontsikh and A. V. Aponchuk *Izv. Vyssh. Uchebn. Zaved. Svetn. Metal*, 1987, 1, 117.
12. C. D. Hewitt, K. Winborne, D. Margrey, J. R. P. Nicholson, M. G. Savory, J. Savory and M. R. Wills, *Clin. Chem.* (in press).
13. W. Slavin, *J. Anal. Atomic Spect.*, 1986, 1, 281.
14. S. Brown, R. L. Bertholf, M. R. Wills and J. Savory, *Clin. Chem.*, 1984, 30, 1216.
15. F. Y. Leung and A. R. Henderson, *Clin. Chem.*, 1982, 28, 2139.
16. M. Bettinelli, U. Baroni, F. Fontana and P. Poisetti, *Analyst*, 1985, 110, 19.
17. M. D. Tonge and J. P. Day, *2nd Nordic Symposium on Trace Elements in Human Health and Diseases*, 1987, Odense, Denmark (Abstract H2).
18. B. V. L'vov, V. G. Nikolaev, E. A. Norman, L. K. Polizik and M. Mojica, *Spectrochim. Acta*, 1986, 41B, 1043.
19. D. C. Baxter and W. Frech, *Spectrochim. Acta*, 1987, 42B, 1005.
20. J. Declina, *Anal. Chem.*, 1982, 54, 2097.
21. C. Boampong, I. D. Brindle, X. Le, L. Pidwerbesky and C. M. C. Ponzoni, *Anal. Chem.*, 1988, 60, 1185.
22. J. W. Hershey and P. N. Keliher, *Spectrochim. Acta Part B*, 1986, 41B, 713.
23. B. J. Jones, B. W. Smith and J. D. Winefordner, *Anal. Chem.*, 1989, 61, 1670.
24. L. J. Moore and L. A. Machlan, *Anal. Chem.*, 1972, 44, 2291.
25. M. A. Klienick, D. J. Frederickson and W. I. Manton, *Anal. Chem.*, 1983, 55, 921. 26. M. B. Rabinowitz, *Biol. Trace Elemen. Res.*, 1987, 12, 223.
27. A. L. Yergey, N. E. Vieira and D. G. Covell, *Biomed. Environ. Mass Spectrom.*, 1987, 14, 603.
28. J. D. Turnlund, *Biol. Trace Elemen. Res.*, 1987, 12, 247.

29. A. L. Gray, Proc. Soc. Anal. Chem., 1974, 11, 182.
30. A. L. Gray and A. R. Date, Analyst, 1983, 1033.
31. A. L. Gray, Spectrochim. Acta, 1986, 41B, 151.
32. T. D. B. Lyon, G. S. Fell, R. C. Hutton and A. N. Eaton, J. Anal. Atom. Spectrom., 1988, 58, 1334.
33. R. E. Serfass, J. J. Thompson and R. S. Houk, Anal. Chim. Acta, 1986, 188, 73.
34. C. Veillon, W. R. Wolf and B. E. Guthrie, Anal. Chem., 1979, 51, 1022.
35. K. W. M. Siu, M. E. Bednas and S. S. Berman, Anal. Chem., 1983, 55, 473.
36. D. C. Reamer and C. Veillon, Anal. Chem., 1981, 53, 2166.
37. W. Schafer and K. Ballschmiter, Fresenious' Z. Anal. Chem., 1983, 315, 475.
38. D. D. Miller and D. Van Campen, Am. J. Clin. Nutr., 1979, 32, 2354.
39. P. E. Johnson, J. Nutr., 1982, 112, 1414.
40. D. L. Hachey, J. C. Blais and P. D. Klein, Anal. Chem., 1980, 52, 1131.
41. B. A. Davis, K. S. Hui, D. A. Durden and A. A. Boulton, Biomed. Mass Spectrom., 1976, 3, 71.
42. W. T. Buckley, S. N. Hucklin, J. J. Budac and G. K. Elgendorf, Anal. Chem., 1982, 54, 504.
43. B. R. Kowalski, T. L. Isenhour and R. E. Sievers, Anal. Chem., 1969, 41, 998.
44. S. K. Aggarwal, M. Kinter, M. R. Wills, J. Savory and D. A. Herold, Anal. Chim. Acta, 1989, 224, 83.
45. S.K. Aggarwal, M. Kinter, M. R. Wills, J. Savory and D. A. Herold, Anal. Chem.,1989, 61, 1099.
46. S. K. Aggarwal, M. Kinter, M. R. Wills, J. Savory and D. A. Herold, Anal. Chem., 1990, 62, 111.
47. R. A. Felder, J. C. Boyd, J. Savory, K. Margrey, A. Martinez and D. Vaughn, Persp. on Clin. Lab. Automation, 1988, 8, 699.
48. D. M. Smith Jr., J.A. Pitcock, and W. M. Murphy, Am. J. Clin. Pathol., 1982, 77, 341.
49. D. P. Perl, D. C. Gajdusek, R. M. Garruto, R. T. Yanagihara, and C. J. Gibbs, Jr., Science, 1982, 217, 1053.
50. B. J. Boyce, H. Y. Elder, G. S. Fell, W. A. P. Nicholson, G. D. Smith, D. W. Dempster, C. C. Gray, and I. T. Boyle, Scanning Electron Microsc., 1981, 111, 29.
51. G. Cournot-Witmer, J. Zingraff, J. J. Plachot, F. Escaig, R. Lefevre, P. Boumati, A. Bourdeau, M. Garabedian, P. Galle, R. Bourdon, T. Drueke, and S. Balsan, Kidney Int. 1981, 20, 375.
52. P. Galle, J. P. Berry and S. Duckett, Acta Neuropathol. 1980, 49, 245.
53. M. E. De Broe, F. L. Van de Vyver, A. B. Bekaert, P. D'Haese, G. J. Paulus, W. J. Visser, R. Van Grieken, F. A. de Wolff, and A. H. Verbueken, In: Trace Elements in Renal Insufficiency; E. A. Quellhorst, K. Finke, C. Fuchs, Eds.; Basel:Karger, 1983, 37.

54. A. H. Verbueken, F. L. Van de Vyver, R. E. Van Grieken, G. J. Paulus, E. F. Visser, P. D'Haese, M. E. De Broe, Clin Chem. 1984, 30, 763.
55. D. Vandeputte, J. Savory, R. E. Van Grieken, W. A. Jacob, R. L. Bertholf, and M. R. Wills, Biomed. Environ. Mass Spectrom. 1989, 18, 598.
56. M. Isaacson, Scanning Electron Microscopy, 1978, 1, 763.
57. F. P. Ottensmeyer, and J. W. Andrew, J. Ultrastructure Res. 1980, 72, 336.
58. D. F. Vandeputte, R. E. Van Grieken, J. Savory, M. R. Wills, and W. A. Jacob, 1st European Workshop on Modern Developments and Applications in Microbeam Analysis (Abstract). Antwerp, Belgium, 8-10 March 1989.
59. A. Aitio, and J. Järvisalo, Pure Appl. Chem. 1984, 56, 549.
60. H. G. Seiler, In: Handbook on Toxicity of Inorganic Compounds, H. G. Seiler, H. Sigel, Eds.; New York: Marcel Dekker, Inc., 1988, 39.
61. S. S. Brown, S. Nomoto, M. Stoeppler, and F. W. Sunderman, Jr. Pure Appl. Chem. 1981, 53, 773.
62. J. Savory, and M. R. Wills, In: Aluminium and Health A Critical Review, H. J. Gitelman, Ed.; New York: Marcel Dekker, Inc., 1988, 1.
63. J. R. Moody, and E. S. Beary, Talanta, 1982, 29, 1003.
64. J. H. Mattinson, Anal. Chem., 1972, 44, 1715.
65. R. P. Maas, and S. A. Dressing, Anal. Chem., 1982, 55, 808.
66. F. W. Sunderman, C. Crisostomo, M. C. Reid, S. M. Hopfer, and S. Nomoto, Ann. Clin. Lab. Sci., 1984, 14, 232.
67. S. Brown, R. L. Bertholf, M. R. Wills, and J. Savory, Clin. Chem., 1984, 30, 1216.
68. S. Brown, N. Mendoza, R. L. Bertholf, R. Ross, M. R. Wills, and J. Savory, Res. Commun. Chem. Pathol. Pharmacol., 1986, 53, 105.
69. J. R. P. Nicholson, M. G. Savory, J. Savory, and M. R. Wills, Clin. Chem., 1989, 35, 488.

Principal Components Analysis for the Determination of Ni in Urine by ICP-MS

Douglas M. Templeton and Margaret-Anne Vaughan

DEPARTMENT OF CLINICAL BIOCHEMISTRY, UNIVERSITY OF TORONTO, TORONTO, CANADA M5G 1L5

1 INTRODUCTION

In common with a number of elements of the first transition series, the determination of Ni in biological fluids continues to be a challenge[1]. Only recently can we place some confidence in reported concentrations of Ni in human serum[2]. Largely due to the efforts of Sunderman's lab[3,4], a value of about 0.2 - 0.3 µg/L appears accurate. This value has been set using Zeeman-corrected electrothermal atomic absorption spectrometry. Detection limits for this technique are presently in the 0.05 - 0.1 µg/L range[5,6]. An alternative to electrothermal atomic absorption for Ni analysis remains elusive. An ideal approach would allow measurement of minute quantities of biological samples, would have detection limits for Ni at the 0.1 µg/L level or better, would require minimal sample processing (thus reducing opportunities for sample aldulteration), and would be capable of yielding isotope information. An important contribution to Ni isotope analysis has been made by Aggarawal et al.[7]. They have reported isotope dilution analysis of National Institute of Standards and Technology (Gaithersburg, MD)(NIST) freeze dried urine by gas chromatography-mass spectrometry (GC-MS). Using ^{62}Ni enrichment, independent measurements of 83.7 ± 2.2 and 79.6 ± 2.9 µg/L of Ni were determined (recommended value of 70 µg/L)[7]. A sensitivity down to the µg/L level was reported. Disadvantages of the published GC-MS method include the need to digest and evaporate the sample, perform chemical synthesis of organic chelates of Ni, and analyse the chelates after separation by gas chromatography. Here we describe an approach for determining Ni that circumvents some of these problems. A major objective of our work is to facilitate stable isotope tracer studies in human subjects. We have chosen urine as a test fluid because its high Ca content makes it an exceptionally difficult matrix for ICP-MS, and because of the importance of urinary Ni for monitoring exposure in a non-invasive manner in the workplace[8].

Advantages and Disadvantages of ICP-MS

In the ICP-MS experiment, a sample is aspirated into an inductively coupled argon plasma and the plasma is sampled by a quadrupole mass filter to determine its ion composition. Following the pioneering work of Gray with a d.c. plasma[9], several technological advances allowed commercialization of the instrumentation during the first half of the last decade (see [10] for a comprehensive review of the history, theory and performance of ICP-MS). Advantages to the approach include ease of sample introduction, and the implicit provision of isotope information. Detection limits for Ni are about 0.03 µg/L with present instrumentation[11]. Furthermore, rapid peak hopping with typical dwell times of 1 s or less allows rapid sequential multielement analysis. Nevertheless, spectral interferences in the mass range of the Ni isotopes create hitherto unsolved problems for the analysis of most complex matrices.

The mass spectral interferences seen in ICP-MS are of three general types. Atomic isobaric interferences arise when one or more additional elements have naturally occurring isotopes of the same mass as the analyte isotope. If isobaric interferences are present in the sample, the analyst may seek another isotope of the analyte for observation. Alternatively, one may measure another isotope of the interfering ion that is itself free from interference, and then apply a correction based on the known natural abundances of the interferent isotopes. Polyatomic ions are a second cause of mass overlap, since the combination of two or more atoms can produce the same mass (to within accessible resolution) as the analyte. The origin of the polyatomic ions is not well understood. Perhaps they arise in the plasma itself, during expansion into the vacuum, or at the boundary layer along the sampler cone. Finally, doubly charged ions of an atom with twice the mass of the analyte give rise to a signal at the same mass-to-charge (m/z) ratio as the singly charged analyte. For example, both $^{130}Ba^{++}$ and $^{65}Cu^+$ are observed at a m/z ratio of 65. The occurrence of doubly charged ions is a minor event, and generally significant only for elements with low second ionization potentials (e.g. Ba, Ca). Isobaric, polyatomic and doubly charged ion interferences are more problematic below mass 80 (the $^{40}Ar^+$ dimer), and present a challenge in the analysis of many lighter elements, including Ni, by ICP-MS. They have been extensively investigated by Horlick and coworkers.[12,13]

Ni Analysis by ICP-MS

While the analysis of Ni in standard solutions and most inorganic reference materials by ICP-MS presents no special difficulties, more complex biological matrices (containing Fe, Zn and Ca) are problematic. Several isobaric and polyatomic interferences with Ni isotopes

Table 1 Spectral Interferences in the Region of the Ni Isotopes

MASS	ELEMENT	INTERFERENCES
56	Fe(91.66)[a]	^{40}ArO, ^{40}CaO
57	Fe(2.19)	^{40}AroH, ^{40}CaOH
58	**Ni(67.77)**, Fe(0.33)	^{42}CaO, NaCl
59	Co(100)	^{43}CaO, ^{42}CaOH
60	Ni(26.16)	^{43}CaOH, ^{44}CaO
61	**Ni(1.25)**	^{44}CaOH
62	**Ni(3.66)**	^{46}CaO, Na$_2$O, NaK
63	Cu(69.1)	^{46}CaOH, ^{40}ArNa
64	**Ni(1.16)**, Zn(48.89)	^{32}SO$_2$, ^{32}S$_2$, ^{48}CaO
65	Cu(30.9)	^{33}S^{32}S, ^{33}SO$_2$, ^{48}CaOH

[a] Natural abundances in parentheses.

are given in Table 1, along with the abundances of all the natural isotopes of Ni. Even when isobaric corrections are applied, the presence of Fe in biological materials generally precludes analysis of Ni at m/z = 58. Similarly, ^{64}Ni is obscured by the major isotope of Zn. This leaves ^{60}Ni as the isotope of choice for total Ni determination, with ^{61}Ni and ^{62}Ni available for isotope dilution and tracer studies. However, Ca oxide and hydroxide formation in the ICP potentially interferes with all Ni isotopes. In particular, the high Ca content of urine (typically 200 mg/L) raises difficulties, and the interesting comment has been made that "the chemical composition of urine is such that it favours the formation of polyatomic ions"[14]. Nevertheless, several successful analyses of biological samples have been reported.

Nickel (23 μg/L) was successfully determined in a lobster hepatopancreas digest with ICP-MS[15]. This is somewhat surprising, as the Ni measurement was performed at mass 58, and the solution was expected to contain 1.9 mg/L of Fe. Presumably isobaric corrections for ^{58}Fe were applied, based on measurement of ^{57}Fe. McLaren and co-workers have used standard addition and isotope dilution to measure Ni in several marine reference materials[16-18]. Mass discrimination was reported for the ratios 61/60 and 62/60, compared to the IUPAC expected natural abundances, and corrections of 1.060 and 1.129, respectively, were at first applied[16], and then later abandoned[17]. Determination of Ni in an open ocean water reference material, NASS-2, by isotope dilution ICP-MS using the 62/60 ratio required a 50-fold pre-concentration[17]. Standard addition was found superior to isotope dilution for the analysis of Ni in tissue digests[18]. Significant overlap of ^{63}Cu with ^{62}Ni at low resolution (1.1 amu) was overcome at higher resolution, but 62/60 ratios remained lower, and 61/60 ratios higher, than in inorganic standard solutions, on account of CaO and CaOH formation. Thus polyatomic and isobaric interferences, as well as probable mass discrimination, have impeded development of a generally applicable technique for the determination of Ni in biological samples by ICP-MS.

2 MATERIALS AND METHODS

^{62}Ni (found 94.85 %) was obtained from Oak Ridge National Laboratory as Ni powder and was dissolved in HNO_3 (Suprapur; Merck). Stock solutions of elemental standards were from SPEX Industries (St. Laurent, Quebec). Standard Reference Material No. 2670 (Trace Elements in Urine) was from NIST and was reconstituted with 20.0 mL deionized water according to the supplier's instructions.

All analyses were done using a Perkin Elmer Sciex Elan 250 ICP-MS. The extended torch supplied with the instrument was positioned such that the tip of the Cu sampler was 20 mm from the end of the load coil. A Tylan F2-280 mass flow controller was used to control the inner gas flow rate. Samples were analysed as aqueous solutions nebulized through a Meinhard nebulizer into a Scott spray chamber. Rhodium (0.1 mg/L) was used as an internal standard. No corrections for isobaric overlap were applied at the time of measurement. Data were acquired in multielement mode at low resolution. Operating conditions for the ICP-MS are given in Table 2.

Table 2 ICP-MS Operating Conditions

R.F. forward power	1.3 kW	Measurement time	5 s
		Dwell time	50 ms
Gas flow rates		Repeats	5
outer	12 L/min	Points per peak	3
intermediate	2 L/min		
inner	1 L/min		
Ion lenses			
	Bessel box barrel		4.2
	plates		-11.4 V
	photon stop		-6.4V
	Einzel		-16.4 V

Principal Components Analysis

Although principal component analysis (PCA) has not found widespread application by the biological trace element community, it has proven useful in areas of chemistry such as spectrophotometry and mass spectrometry. It can be applied whenever a measurement can be expressed as a linear sum of product terms, as for example a signal intensity arising from several independent species. Thus in ICP-MS, when PCA is applied for the purpose of resolving spectral overlaps, each principal component is associated with one of the species contributing to the measured signals. If measurements are made at n masses, these define a mass hyperspace of dimension n, whose coordinate axes are identified with each mass. These axes are transformed into a set of n mutually orthogonal eigenvectors that are associated with the variance in the data. If these are ordered by decreasing eigenvalue, the first eigenvector spans the maximum variance in the data, the second the next greatest variance, and so on. Each spectrum appears as a unique point in mass space, and transforms to a point in

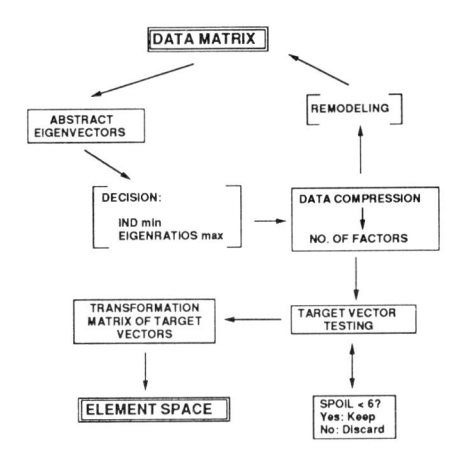

Figure 1 Algorithm used for PCA of Ni

eigenvector space. At this stage, the number of eigenvectors necessary to reproduce the data matrix to within experimental error is found. This represents the number of components in the system. Rejection of lower eigenvalues eliminates some random error from the measurements and compresses the eigenvector space to lower dimension. The remaining principal components carry residual error that cannot be removed by further analysis. In order to identify these components with elements, it is necessary to transform the compressed eigenvector space into element space. In element space, each axis corresponds to an element and the vector components of the point corresponding to the original spectrum in mass space explicitly represent the signal arising from each element. This procedure is outlined in Fig. 1. For a fuller description of these procedures, the interested reader is referred to the book by Malinowski and Howery[19].

In the present study, these transformations were carried out using Matlab™ on a Macintosh SE/30 microcomputer. Data from r independent spectral measurements at c different masses were placed in a r x c data matrix [D] and the covariance matrix $[Z] = [D]^T[D]$ calculated. PCA was done using the NIPALs method[20]. If the experimental error is known with good precision, it can be used to decide the number of principal components to be kept. Here the decision was made empirically. The eigenvectors with the larger eigenvalues are associated primarily with the data and those with the smaller values primarily represent error. We have used two criteria to decide the cutoff between the eigenvectors representing the data and the error, the IND function of Malinowski and Howery[19] and successive eigenratios as employed by Wirsz and Blades[21]. IND is an empirical function of the residual standard deviation that reaches a minimum when calculated with the number of eigenvectors describing the data. The second approach assumes that the ratio between successive eigenvalues is a maximum at the number of principal components, and decreases for eigenvalues associated primarily with error. The rotation into element space was accomplished by target transformation. In this approach, a set of independent test vectors that covers the eigenvector space is used to construct the transformation matrix. These arise from the independent mass spectra of each component, usually single element standards. If the test vectors are good (i.e. if the standard elements are true components of the sample) they will not introduce excess error. Otherwise, they will spoil the system. An indicator function SPOIL[19] was used to provide a measure of the appropriateness of the test vector. Target vectors were retained when SPOIL < 6. When the full set of target vectors was found, a transformation matrix composed of them was used to accomplish the rotation into element space and calculate the target factors. Each axis in hyperspace was identified with an element and projected onto the element axis to obtain relative concentrations. Finally, the actual concentration of each element was obtained by multiplying the target factors by the concentration of the appropriate target standard.

3   RESULTS AND DISCUSSION

A mass scan of any simple biological matrix in the region m/z = 58-64 reveals ratios of signal intensities quite different from those expected for the isotopes of Ni, even when corrections for monoisotopic interferences (^{58}Fe, ^{64}Zn) are applied. Polyatomic interferences are expected (Table 2) and point to Ca as a problematic concomitant when Ni is to be analyzed. Addition of 16 (oxide) or 17 (hydroxide) mass units to the significant isotopes of Ca reproduces the masses of all the naturally occurring Ni isotopes.

<u>Oxide Suppression</u>

The elements of the first transition series lie in a particularly busy region of the ICP mass spectrum; additional, previously unidentified interferences are likely. Nevertheless, the expected prominance of oxide interferences with Ni led us to evaluate the usefulness of oxide suppression. The mechanism of oxide formation in ICP-MS is poorly understood, but oxides may arise in the boundary layer along the sampler cone. The effect of instrument parameter settings on analyte signals in ICP-MS has been studied in detail[10,22,23]. The R.F. forward power, central gas flow rate and ion sampling depth all have an effect on the signal levels. Commonly the behaviour of a signal is characterized by a plot of intensity against central gas flow rate. This typically shows a maximum, and similar behaviour is observed for oxide and hydroxide species. However, it has been shown that under some circumstances, oxides and hydroxides have maxima at higher flow rates than singly charged analyte ions. By operating at reduced central gas flow rates, these interferences were minimized with earlier instrumentation[13].

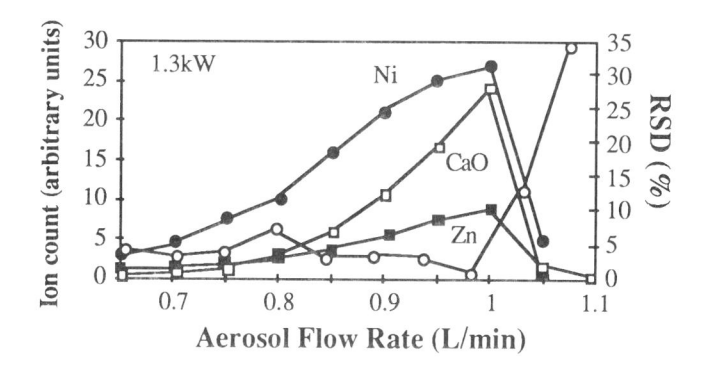

Figure 2 Dependence of the intensity of Ni, Zn and CaO Signals on central gas flow rate at an R.F. power of 1.3 kW. —o— shows the relative standard deviation (RSD) of the Zn signal.

Improvements to current ICP-MS instrumentation, particularly to the ion optics, have largely eliminated the separation between the maxima of M^+, MO^+ and MOH^+ species. When the parameter behaviour was investigated for the present study, signals of CaO, CaOH and Zn reached maxima at the same flow rates, for all values of R. F. power and sampling depth tested. Ca and Zn were not observed together because of the overlap problem. CaO (m/z=56) and ^{66}Zn were observed in one solution, and ^{58}Ni and ^{66}Zn in another. All species reached maximum signal intensity at the same flow rate, which yielded the lowest relative standard deviation (Fig. 2). Consequently, the CaO and CaOH interferences on Ni cannot be separated by this approach.

Principal Components Analysis

Intensity data were acquired at m/z = 58, 60, 61 and 62 for solutions of 3 to 30 µg/L Ni in 0, 40 or 100 mg/L Ca. PCA appropriately identified the presence of two components, and based on target vectors of Ca and Ni standards, separated the two signals and correctly reproduced the data. Therefore, we proceeded to analyse the urine reference material.

Urine was diluted to 40% and analyzed at the same four masses as above (Table 3). The suggested level of Ni pending certification in this material is 70 µg/L. First Ni was determined by standard addition using the unprocessed data at both m/z = 58 and 62. The result was in error by 10% at m/z = 58 due to the presence of ^{42}CaO. At m/z = 62, the error was 86%, probably due to additional Na species (vide infra). A two component system was used with and without combined standard addition, and gave acceptable results in each case. However, remodelling of the raw data, although acceptable at masses 58, 60 and 61, was about 40% too low at m/z = 62. This is consistent with the large error when the raw data were used at this mass, and demonstrates that if isotopic profiles are to be obtained, additional interferences must be considered. Solutions of urea, NaCl and KCl, at levels typically found in urine, were analysed singly and in combination. The NaCl/KCl solution (1 g/L Na, 0.5 g/L K) had intensities at m/z = 62, arising from ^{23}Na^{39}K and Na$_2$O, as well as a moderate signal at m/z = 58 from ^{23}Na^{35}Cl. When this solution was added as a target vector in a 3-component analysis, data remodelling was successful at all four masses (not shown), and the suggested level of Ni was obtained (Table 3).

Table 3 Ni in SRM 2670 "Trace Metals in Urine" determined by several methods. The suggested value is 70 µg/L.

Method	Standard addition	m/z	[Ni](µg/L) (± 1sd)
Raw data	Yes	58	77 ± 1
Raw data	Yes	62	130 ± 1
PCA (2-component)	No	58,60,61,62	69
PCA (2-component)	Yes	58,60,61,62	72 ± 1
PCA (3-component	Yes	58,60,61,62	69 ± 1

Isotopic Separation

Separation of isotopically distinct sources of Ni in a urine sample presents an additional complication in that, treating the two Ni sources as distinct components, a 4-component analysis (2 Ni, Ca and NaK) should be required. Because the system must be overdetermined in PCA[19], a fifth mass must be analyzed. This must be relevant without introducing any additional components. Inspection of Table 1 shows that choices are limited. However, only Co and Ca species are found at m/z = 59, and because the concentration of Co in urine is normally very low, this mass was added. Urine from healthy volunteers with no measurable Ni was spiked with both naturally abundant and ^{62}Ni-enriched Ni solutions. Three-component PCA (Ni, ^{62}Ni, Ca) gave reasonable results,

Table 4 Analysis by PCA of Naturally Abundant Ni and Enriched ^{62}Ni in a Urine Matrix

Concentration (µg/L)		Measured (µg/L) 3 components		Measured (µg/L) 4 components	
Ni(na)[a]	Ni(en)[b]	Ni(na)	Ni(en)	Ni(na)	Ni(e)
20	10	22	12	22	11
20	6	20	7	19	6
10	10	12	10	10	10
10	6	12	7	12	6

[a] Naturally abundant Ni
[b] Ni enriched in ^{62}Ni.

although an improvement was gained at lower concentrations when a fourth component (NaCl/KCl) was added (Table 4). This is to be expected, because the enriched spike was at the mass of NaK. In this worst case, the 4-component analysis of urine, the limits of detection for Ni were estimated to be 1 µg/L.

4 SUMMARY

Anlysis of Ni in biological fluids by ICP-MS is feasible when corrections for Ca species and other minor interferents are applied. PCA is successful in this regard, allowing analysis of Ni in urine, and achieving separation of isotopically spiked Ni in this Ca-rich matrix.

5 ACKNOWLEDGEMENT

This work was supported by grants from the Ni Producers Environmental Research Association (NiPERA) and the Province of Ontario (U.R.I.F.), and by contributions from the M.D.S. Health Group.

6 REFERENCES.

1. M. Stoeppler, In 'Nickel in the Human Environment, (F.W. Sunderman Jr, ed.), IARC Scientific Publications, Lyon, No. 53, 1984, p. 459.
2. J. Versieck and R. Cornelis, 'Trace Elements in Human Plasma and Serum', CRC Press, Boca Raton, Florida, 1989, p. 72.
3. C. N. Leach Jr, J. V. Linden, S. M. Hopfer, M. C. Crisostomo and F. W. Sunderman Jr, Clin. Chem., 1985, 31, 556.
4. J. V. Linden, S. M. Hopfer, H. R. Grossling and F. W. Sunderman Jr, Ann. Clin. Lab. Sci., 1985, 15, 459.
5. F. W. Sunderman Jr, M. C. Crisostomo, M. C. Reid, S. M. Hopfer and S. Nomoto, Ann.Clin.Lab.Sci., 1984, 14, 232.

6. J. R. Andersen, B. Gammelgaard and S. Reimert, Analyst, 1986, 111, 721.
7. S. K. Aggarawal, M. Kinter, M. R. Wills, J. Savory and D. A. Herold, Anal.Chem., 1989, 61, 1099.
8. F. W. Sunderman Jr, In 'Handbook on Toxicity of Inorganic Compounds' (H.G. Seiler and H. Sigel, eds.) Marcel Dekker, New York, 1988, p. 453.
9. A. L. Gray, Analyst, 1975, 100, 289.
10. R. S. Houk and J. J. Thompson, Mass Spectrom. Rev., 1988, 7, 425.
11. D. Templeton, A. Paudyn and A. Baines, Biol. Trace Elem. Res., 1989, 22, 17.
12. S. H. Tan and G. Horlick, Appl. Spectrosc., 1986, 40, 445.
13. M. A. Vaughan and G. Horlick, Appl. Spectrosc., 1986, 40, 434.
14. T. D. B. Lyon, G. S. Fell, R. C. Hutton and A. N. Eaton, J. Anal. At. Spectrom., 1988, 3, 265.
15. P. S. Ridout, H. R. Jones and J. G. Williams, Analyst, 1988, 113, 1383.
16. D. Beauchemin, J. W. McLaren, A. P. Mykytiuk and S. S. Berman, J. Anal. At. Spectrom., 1988, 3, 305.
17. D. Beauchemin, J. W. McLaren and S. S. Berman, J. Anal. At. Spectrom., 1988, 3, 775.
18. D. Beauchemin, J. W. McLaren, S. N. Willie and S. S. Berman, Anal. Chem., 1988, 60, 687.
19. E. R. Malinowski and D. G. Howery, 'Factor Analysis in Chemistry', John Wiley and Sons, New York, N.Y., 1980.
20. P. Geladi and B. R. Kowalski, Anal. Chim. Acta, 1986, 185, 1.
21. D. F. Wirsz and M. W. Blades, Anal. Chem., 1986, 58, 51.
22. M. A. Vaughan, G. Horlick and S. H. Tan, J. Anal. Atom. Spectrom., 1987, 2, 765.
23. G. Horlick, S. H. Tan, M. A. Vaughan and C. A. Rose, Spectrochim. Acta, 1985, 40B, 1555.

Atomic Fluorescence Spectrometry for the Determination of Mercury in Biological Samples

G. Vermeir, C. Vandecasteele*, and R. Dams

LABORATORY OF ANALYTICAL CHEMISTRY, UNIVERSITY OF GENT, INSTITUTE FOR NUCLEAR SCIENCES, PROEFTUINSTRAAT 86, B - 9000 GENT, BELGIUM

1 INTRODUCTION

Atomic fluorescence spectrometry has frequently been applied for the analysis of water samples[1,2]. For several interesting biological samples direct analysis is possible[3,4], but this is not the case for very low concentrations as for example those encountered in milk powder or serum. Preconcentration on a gold absorber can be applied.

This paper describes the optimization of a commercial system for the analysis of biological samples for mercury by atomic fluorescence spectrometry with and without preconcentration on gold. The accuracy was assessed by analysing several certified reference materials. Additionally, hair and urine samples were analysed and the results compared to literature values.

2 EXPERIMENTAL

Reagents

All chemicals were reagent grade and Millipore MilliQ water was used throughout. A standard stock solution of mercury (1.000 g/L) was prepared by dissolving mercury (II) oxide in 14 mol/L nitric acid and diluting to 1 L. Working standard solutions (ng/L range) were prepared daily by dilution immediately before use. All standards, blank and sample solutions were stable for up to 10 hours using 2% nitric acid (v/v). The stannous chloride solution was prepared by dissolving 20 g of the dihydrate (highest purity, UCB) in 80 mL of boiling 12 mol/L hydrochloric acid followed by dilution with 200 mL of water and 600 mL of 1.5 mol/L sulfuric acid. This solution was cooled and purged for 30 min with nitrogen.

---

* Research Director of the Belgian National Fund for Scientific Research

Dissolution Procedure

100 mg of solid sample or 10 mL of liquid sample was weighed directly into a Teflon PFA (perfluoroalkoxy) digestion vessel and subboiled concentrated nitric acid (1 mL for the solid samples and 5 mL for the liquid samples) was added. Six sealed vessels and a beaker filled with 50 mL of water, to absorb excess of microwave energy, were placed inside a plastic box which was closed and put in the microwave oven (Amana, Model R.S. 560A). The dissolution programme consisted of three steps: 20% power for 8 min, 40% power for 8 min and 60% power for 4 min. After cooling, the digest was transferred to a volumetric flask and diluted to 100 mL with water.

Mercury Determination

Direct mercury analysis is carried out using a continuous flow mercury vapour generator (Hydride Generator model No. PSA 10003, PS Analytical, Kemsing, Sevenoaks, England) consisting (Fig 1) of a carrier gas supply; a pumping system delivering a continuous flow of $SnCl_2$ solution, blank and sample; a T-piece where the $SnCl_2$ solution and the blank or the sample are mixed; and a gas/liquid separator devised in house[5]. The sample and blank streams are switched using a combination of two 3 port 2-way miniature Teflon valves as indicated in Fig 1. Blank and samples are pumped at a flow rate of 7 mL/min, $SnCl_2$ is pumped at a flow rate of 3 mL/min.

The batch mercury vapour generation system consists of a reduction aeration cell, a trap with Sn^{2+} solution in KOH and a gold absorber as reported earlier[6]. The mercury collected on the gold absorber is analysed with a two stage desorption unit (Fig 2). The calibration graph is obtained by injecting known amounts of air saturated with mercury vapour. The precision and accuracy of this calibration method and its advantages compared to standard solutions were reported earlier[7].

The atomic fluorescence spectrometer (PS Analytical Merlin Fluorescence detector model no PSA 10023) consists of a high intensity mercury lamp, an open chimney[4] into which the mercury vapour is fed by means of the Ar carrier gas, an interference filter to isolate the 254 nm resonance line and a photodetector. By electronic attenuation, the sensitivity can be adjusted. The response is displayed digitally as a reading from 0 to 199 and as a 0 to 10 mV analog output that can be interfaced to a personal computer or chart recorder.

The analog output is converted to a digital signal by an analog digital convertor. A Tulip personal computer records the time resolved fluorescence signal. Correction of the peak area for baseline drift is possible using time windows, as shown in Fig 3. The system can also be used in the peak height mode.

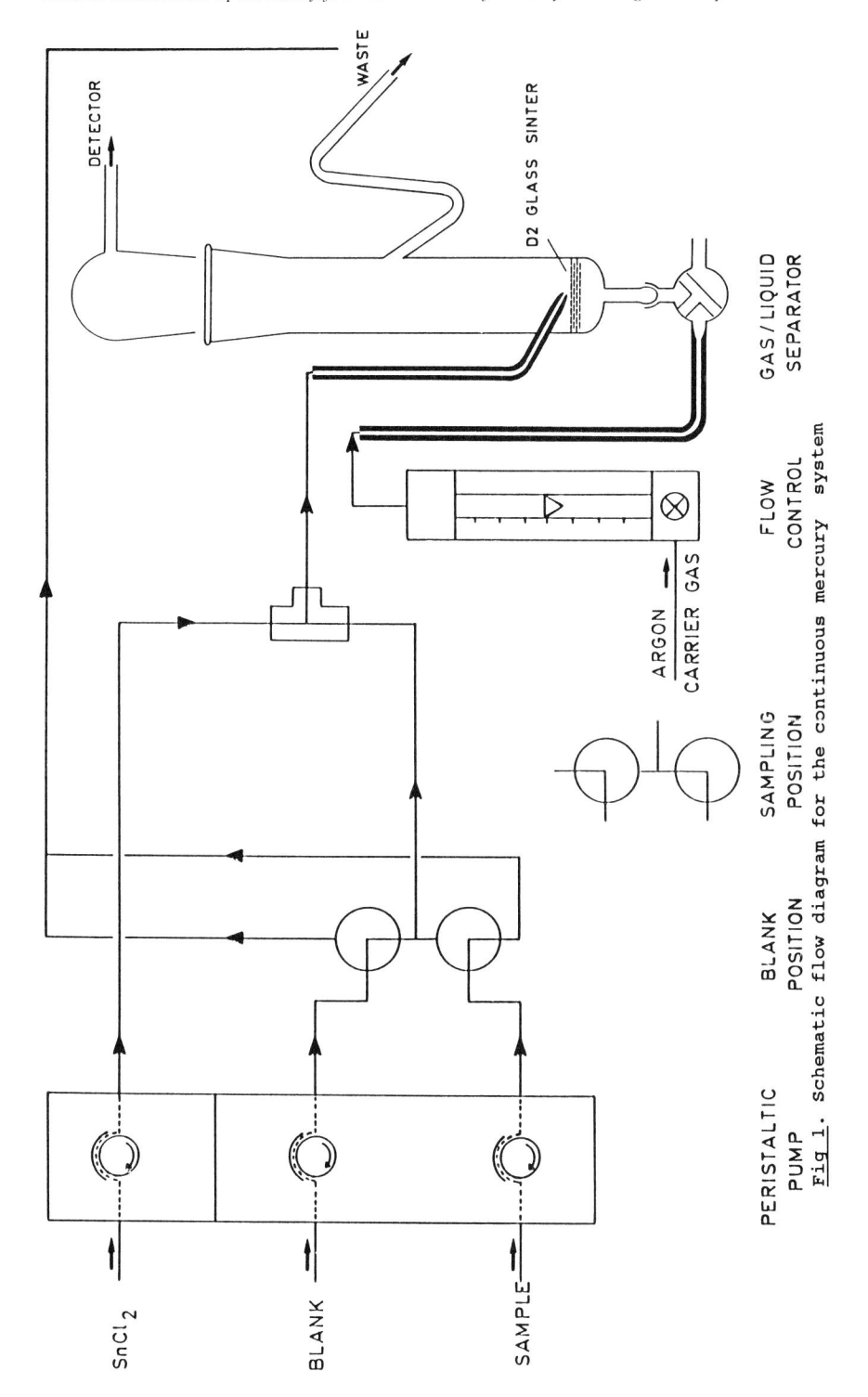

Atomic Fluorescence Spectrometry for Determination of Mercury in Biological Samples   31

Fig 1. Schematic flow diagram for the continuous mercury system

3 RESULTS AND DISCUSSION

The optimized instrumental parameters are given in Table 1. Fig 3 shows the signal output obtained using the direct method and the preconcentration method, indicating that when preconcentration is used the sensitivity is much higher for the same sample volume as a result of the smaller peak width. Table 1 shows the calculation routine for both the continuous mode and the batch mode of operation.

Table 1. Instrumental parameters

	Continuous	Batch
Carrier gas (flow mL/min)	Ar (200)	Ar (500)
Sheath gas	-	-
Sample introduction	1 min 30 s	30 s
Sample volume	7 mL/min	10 mL
$SnCl_2$ concentration	21 g/L	300 g/L
$SnCl_2$ volume	3 mL/min	1 mL
Measuring time	300 s	150 s
Measurements per s	1	2
Integration time	260 s	100 s
Sample introduction time	5-95 s	30-60 s

Detection Limit and Precision

The detection limit defined as the mercury concentration corresponding to three times the standard deviation of the blank, corresponds to 0.9 ng/L and 2 pg respectively. For the continuous mode the precision is generally better than 1 % RSD in the µg/L concentration range and better than 5 % RSD in the ng/L concentration range. For the batch system the precision ranges generally from 5 to 10 %.

Analysis of Reference Materials

In order to verify the accuracy of the two methods, the optimized analytical procedures were used to analyse some certified reference materials (CRM) of the Community Bureau of Reference (BCR) and standard reference materials (SRM) of the National Bureau of Standards (NBS). BCR CRM 151 Milk Powder (spiked); BCR CRM 186 Pig Kidney; BCR RM 397 Human Hair and NBS SRM 1566 Oyster Tissue were analysed directly. For RM 397 we participated in the certification campaign. For NBS SRM 1577 Bovine Liver and BCR CRM 150 Milk Powder, the batch system with preconcentration had to be applied because of the lower mercury level in these samples. The results obtained for the reference materials are given in table 2. For both the continuous system and the batch system good results were obtained.

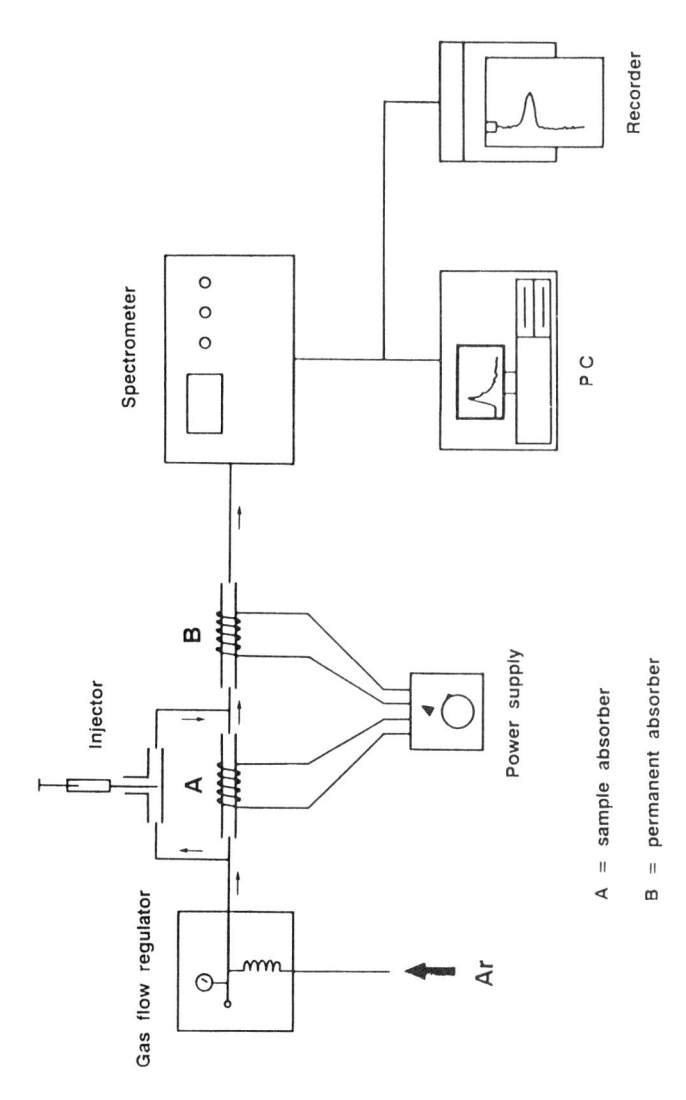

Fig. 2. Analysis set-up for the batch system using preconcentration on a gold absorber

A = sample absorber

B = permanent absorber

Table 2. Analysis of biological reference materials.

Sample	Mercury concentration (ng/g)				
	Found			Certified	
	Mean	SD	N		
CONTINUOUS SYSTEM					
Milk Powder(spiked) BCR CRM 151	102.6	4.8	3	101	± 10
Pig Kidney BCR CRM 186	1987	3	3	1970	± 40
Oyster Tissue NBS SRM 1566	55.6	3.9	3	57	± 15
Human Hair BCR RM 397	11550	240	5	12300	± 900*
BATCH SYSTEM					
Bovine Liver NBS SRM 1577	14.9	2.6	5	16	± 2
Milk Powder(spiked) BCR CRM 150	8.5	1.4	2	9.4	± 1.7

*value proposed for certification.

Determination of Mercury in Human Hair and Urine

Head hair readily incorporates methylmercury at the time the hair is formed[8]. The concentration in newly formed hair is directly proportional to the concentration in the blood. Once incorporated into hair, the concentration remains stable for many years. Providing steps are taken to avoid or remove external contamination, hair forms a record of previous exposure.

The optimized method without preconcentration on gold was used to analyse a hair sample, taken without special precautions to avoid contamination. The mercury concentration in the hair amounts to 1630 ng/g with a standard deviation of 60 ng/g, i.e. within the range given in the literature[9] for non-exposed subjects.

Urine is the chief medium for excretion of inorganic divalent mercury and is most commonly used for biological monitoring. Concentrations in urine probably indicate kidney levels.

The optimized method was used to analyse a urine sample, immediately after collection. The urine sample was analysed both by calibration against aqueous standards and using the standard addition method. The concentrations obtained with the two methods were 4.87 ± 0.02 µg/L and 4.57 ± 0.27 µg/L. The blank for the entire analytical procedure amounts to 13.9 ± 1.0 ng/L and the detection limit to 30 ng/L assuming that a 10 mL

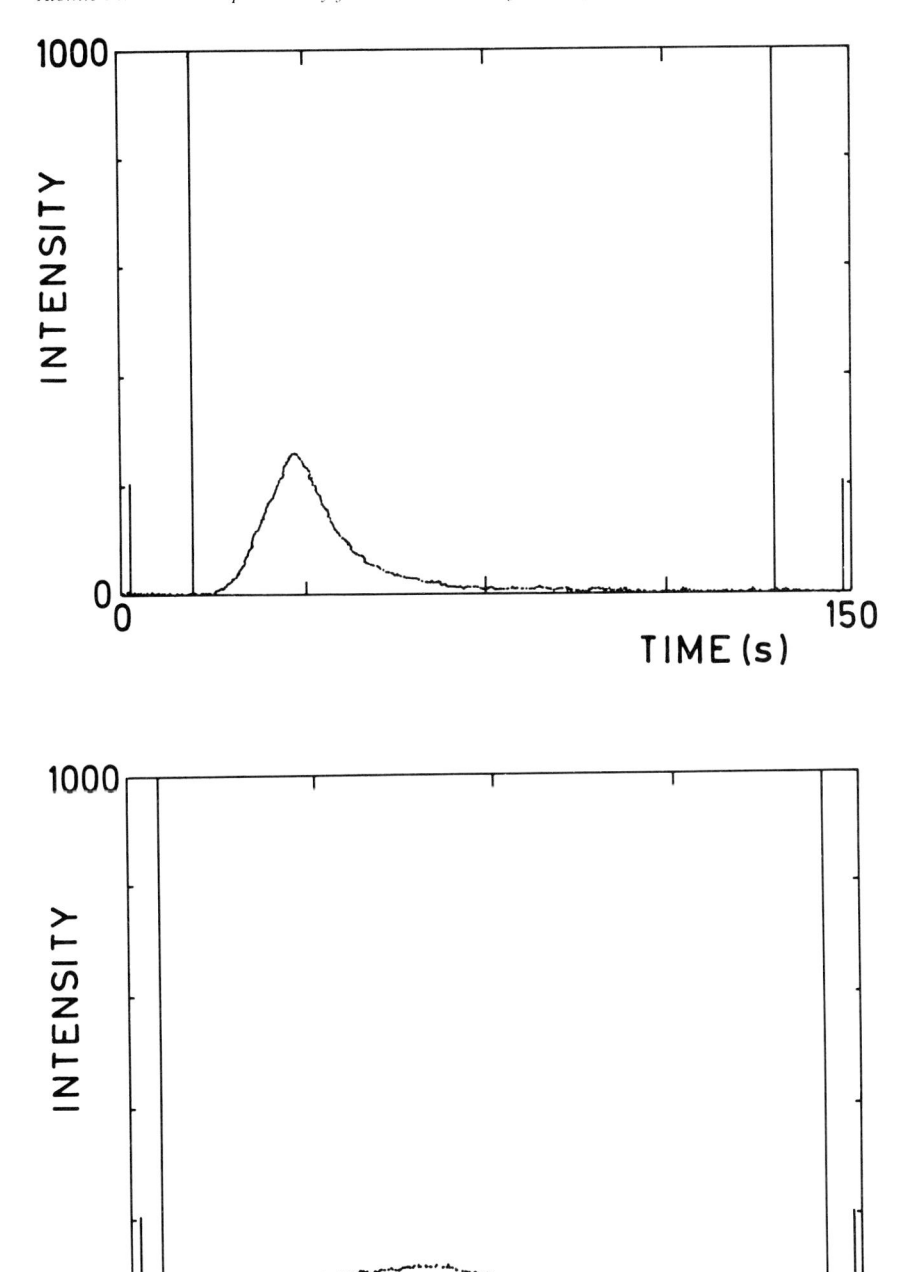

Fig 3. Typical signal output with cursor settings for a 100 pg Hg (top) and a 10 ng Hg/L standard (bottom) introduced at 7 mL/min during 1.5 min.

sample of urine is digested and diluted to 100 mL of which 10 mL is analysed. The concentration found falls within the range for non-exposed subjects[9].

Table 3. Analysis of human hair and urine.

Sample	Mercury concentration			
	Found Mean	SD	n	Literature[9] Range
Hair(ng/g)	1630	60	3	30-4300
Urine(µg/L)	4.87	0.02	3	0.8-6.4

4 CONCLUSION

The determination of mercury in biological samples by atomic fluorescence spectrometry with and without preconcentration on gold is a simple, sensitive and specific method for determining trace and ultra trace levels of mercury. The accuracy is shown by the good agreement between the obtained results and the certified values.

5 REFERENCES

1. K.C. Thompson and G.D. Reynolds, Analyst, 1971, 96, 771.
2. V.I. Muscat and T.J. Vickers, Anal. Chim. Acta, 1971, 57, 23.
3. J.E. Caupeil, P.W. Hendrikx and J.S. Bongres, Anal. Chim. Acta, 1976, 81, 53.
4. K.C. Thompson and R.G. Godden, Analyst, 1975, 100, 544.
5. G. Vermeir, C. Vandecasteele, R. Dams, in preparation.
6. G. Vermeir, C. Vandecasteele, R.Dams, Microchim. Acta, 1988, III, 305.
7. R. Dumarey, E. Temmerman, R. Dams and J. Hoste, Anal. Chim. Acta, 1985, 170, 337.
8. T.W. Clarkson, J. Am. Coll. Toxicol., 1989, 8, Number 7.
9. P. Baron and F. Schweinsberg, Zbl. Hyg., 1989, 188, 84.

Quality Assurance: Achievements, Problems, Prospects

S. S. Brown

WEST MIDLANDS REGIONAL LABORATORY FOR TOXICOLOGY, BIRMINGHAM, B18 7QH, UK

1 INTRODUCTION

The terms "quality assurance" and "quality control" are sometimes used interchangeably in discussions of mandatory clinical laboratory regulations or voluntary accreditation requirements. However, it is helpful[1] to distinguish between two distinct but related features of laboratory performance. *Quality assurance* refers to systems of external requirements placed upon clinical laboratories by governmental agencies or private accreditation organisations. For analyses of trace elements in biological materials, these requirements may be regulatory in nature or voluntary, depending upon the matrix, the medico-legal context and other factors. *Quality control* refers to internal activities undertaken by laboratories to assure that their results are reliable. Quality-control procedures may or may not be required by quality-assurance systems. A third term[1] is also helpful in discussion: *quality ensurance* refers to the appropriate ordering of laboratory tests by clinicians and the correct utilization of laboratory test reports by them. This is the realm of medical decision-making. *Quality* in this case does not refer to the analytical accuracy or precision of the testing process, but to the impact of the testing process on the patient's health care as a function of medical decision-making.

In operational terms, therefore, quality assurance and quality ensurance embrace quality control and quality assessment, and extend beyond them to the early stage of defining the problem or the need, and the late stage of assessing the relevance or usefulness of the analytical result(s). In other words, they encompass - the correct patient (or subject) or population; the correct context; the correct specimen at the correct time; the correct transport and storage; the correct analytical procedure at the correct cost; the correct result and report; the correct interpretation and action; the correct follow-up; the correct writing-up:-

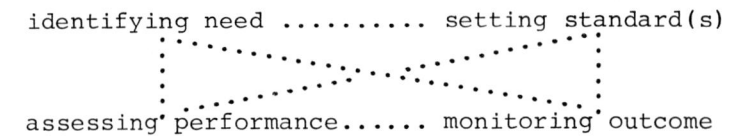

```
       identifying need  .......... setting standard(s)
              ....                        ....
              :   ....              ....     :
              :      ....        ....        :
              :         ....  ....           :
              :          ....                :
              :      ....    ....            :
              :  ....              ....      :
              ....                       ....
       assessing performance ...... monitoring outcome
```

This ideal is easy enough to set out, but it is immensely difficult to put into practice within the framework of trace elements in health and disease. Nevertheless some reasons for the current high level of interest in quality assurance can be outlined as follows:-

a. Good analytical systems for trace element measurements have been available for several decades, but they are expensive both in capital and revenue terms; nowadays value-for-money and quality are all-important criteria in every branch of science, including the medical sciences.

b. In clinical laboratories generally - starting with biochemistry and going on to haematology, microbiology and cytology - the quality of performance has evidently improved over the years; should not the same be true of trace element analysis?

c. The method-dependence of analytical results for trace elements is now well recognised, and with it, the need for a basis of accuracy as well as precision.

d. Modern high-technology industries rely heavily on the use of toxic metals and metaloids. Strong efforts are being made in many countries to protect workers by environmental or biological monitoring - hopefully, recognising the complexities and the implications of physical and chemical speciation.

e. Those trace elements which are of industrial importance in tonnage terms feature strongly in problems of global ecotoxicology. The study of actual or potential adverse health effects, and the consequent legislation which is designed to protect whole populations, need to be supported by measurements which are valid over space and time.

f. Awareness of the essentiality and toxicities of trace elements, and their interactions in vivo, has been a great stimulus to the quantitative analysis of water and foodstuffs, as well as body fluids.

g. Better and more systematic sampling procedures and measurements than hitherto are needed, if there are to be advances in our knowledge of individual or population-based variability, and of the subtleties of chronobiochemistry in trace element metabolism.

What then, has been achieved; what are the problems; and what are the prospects?

2 THE NEED FOR ACCURACY

The general principles of quality assurance of chemical measurements have been authoritatively reviewed and illustrated with regard to: statistical techniques; sampling, measurement and control aspects; reference materials and traceability; audit, validation and reporting.[2] Only a few small details of these important technical issues can be discussed here, but consider first[3] the general needs of the physician or surgeon for high quality - i.e. accurate - test results in diagnosis and treatment:-

a. To conform with published values when there are accepted levels for separating normal from diseased individuals.

b. When there exists a physiological reciprocal relationship between two or more analytes in the same sample.

c. When dosage of medication is predicated on the determined level of some blood constituent.

d. When metabolic exchange studies serve as a guide to diagnosis or treatment.

Each of these desiderata can be illustrated from areas of trace element metabolism or toxicology such as occupational exposure, total parenteral nutrition, deficiency or overload. But how true is the implicit assumption that "published values" are accurate, and if they are accurate, is it valid for the doctor to make comparison with his or her own laboratory's results? It is problematic enough in a single laboratory to be confident that serial results on one patient are meaningful if they extend over 5, 10 or 15 years - calibration materials, techniques and even personnel are sure to change! The practical difficulties are illustrated well by the need for long-term monitoring in occupational or environmental exposure to cadmium[4] or to lead.[5,6] The fact that a certification limit (Figure 1) can be set for suspension from work-related exposure demonstrates of itself the importance of a basis of accuracy in blood lead measurements.[7]

A valuable and wide-ranging commentary on the difficult problem of between-laboratory comparability has been offered.[8] With chromium in human blood, for example, the "normal" concentration has apparently diminished in a log-linear fashion since the introduction of atomic absorption spectroscopy. The marked method-dependency of estimates of "normal" nickel concentrations in human serum/plasma has been pointed out.[9]

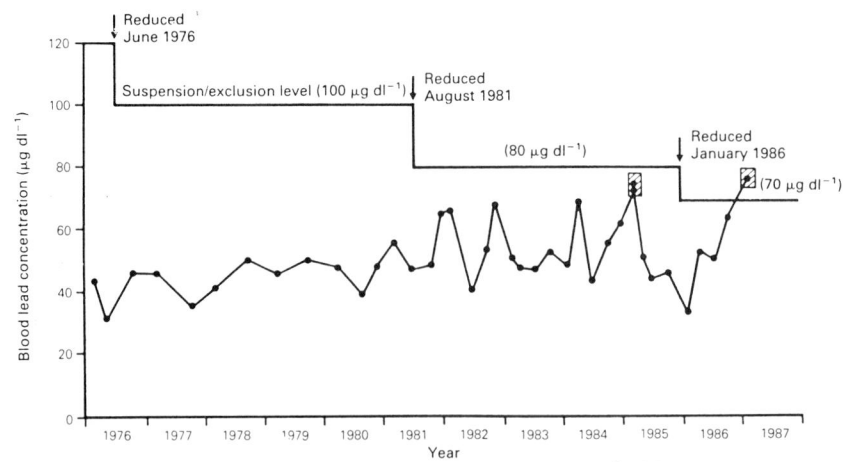

Figure 1 Blood lead concentrations following routine monitoring of occupational lead exposure in one worker over a 12-year period, with two periods of exclusion from exposure. The stepwise reduction in the UK certification limit for male workers is shown (reproduced, with permission, from ref. 6).

Less dramatic, but still very striking anomalies, have been documented for many other trace elements of clinical interest. The underlying reasons are many and varied - inadequate analytical methods, inaccurate calibration, poor laboratory technique in general, lack of statistical control, ignorance of contamination. This last factor has been an important stimulus to the preparation of a human serum pool free of exogeneous contamination.[10] The production, in due course, of baseline reference values for trace element concentrations in this serum will make a very useful contribution to overall assurance of quality in the investigation of "normal" populations. The theory of defining reference values in laboratory medicine generally is well worked out,[11] but the practice in terms of trace elements is difficult. Moreover, is it really feasible to extend this kind of approach to trace elements in the cellular components of blood, to the protein or membrane-bound fractions, or to other body fluids or tissues? What is the physiological and pathophysiological relevance, if any, of the chemical speciation of the trace elements? Is it valid to use "marker" elements, such as gallium for aluminium, lithium for sodium, or strontium for calcium in quantitative metabolic studies? These questions need to be tackled, and serious attempts to do so have been made from time to time. However, the intrinsic difficulties of quality assurance are very great, because the components of a systematic approach[12] to meaningful measurements are largely lacking:-

a. A rational, self-consistent system of units of measurement.

b. The materials to realise in practice the defined units and their derivatives.

c. The availability of accurate methods of measurement based on these reference materials.

d. The transfer of accuracy in space and time, and the validation of "field" methods of analysis, using reference materials and reference methods.

e. Assurance of the long-term integrity of the measurement process.

3 REFERENCE MATERIALS AND METHODS

Reference materials for trace element analyses are important in many fields, and it is useful to distinguish[13] between various types:-

a. Matrix reference materials, which are essentially identical to the actual samples being measured, for example, a defined alloy used in the analysis of steels.

b. Simulated reference materials, which have quite similar properties to the actual samples, for example, an aqueous solution of trace elements used in water analysis.

c. Surrogate reference materials, which have little or no correspondence with the actual samples, for example, a pure chemical used to calibrate the corresponding assay of a serum specimen.

d. Synthetic reference materials, which require the user to carry out a particular operation in order to convert the material into an appropriate form for the actual analysis, such as a gas glow system and a gas permeation tube as used in air pollution analysis.

Trace element reference materials with assigned concentrations have been available for many years in the context of ferrous metallurgy; the market is large, and their commercial impact has been very substantial. The economic forces in respect of biological matrix materials for trace elements are quite different; however, Bowen's kale blazed the trail, followed by the National Bureau of Standards' orchard leaves and liver material. It is very encouraging that clinical laboratories have been willing to put a lot of voluntary effort into cooperative studies such as that which served to characterise the "second generation" reference serum already mentioned,[10] and to assign selenium

Average MRVIS

UK EQAS for Lead in Blood

Average Mean Running Variance Index Score (MRVIS)

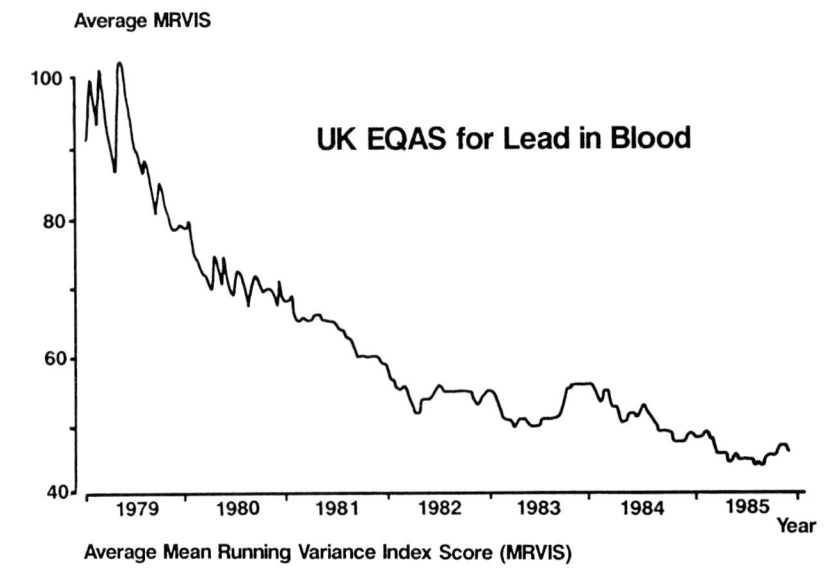

Figure 2 Average Mean Running Variance Index Score (MRVIS), 1979-85, for all participants in the UK National External Quality Assessment Scheme for blood lead analysis (reproduced, with permission, from ref. 17).

concentrations to serum and urine materials with fairly narrow confidence limits.[14] The danger is that these pool materials will deteriorate or be used up before they can be applied to the cross-characterisation of new pools or new analytical methods. More formal cooperative or collaborative campaigns of characterisation have been sponsored by the European Community Bureau of Reference and the International Atomic Energy Agency, which include several kinds of biological matrix materials in their catalogues. But these products are expensive, the range is necessarily limited, and the market for them is likely to remain small in comparison with the analytical needs of high-value/high-volume commerce and industry.

To some extent, therefore, progress has been hindered by a lack of matrix materials with assigned concentrations, but it is encouraging that a recent monograph[15] on trace element analysis explained the importance of reference materials with appropriate matrices. The vital point is that most trace element analysts now recognise the needs not just for good sensitivity and specificity, but also for monitoring repeatability, reproducibility together with other aspects of precision, and inter-laboratory variability.

Proficiency surveys, or external quality assessment schemes, were first introduced into clinical laboratories in the 1940's, following a pattern which had been established by the oils-fats-and-waxes chemists

UK EQAS For Lead in Blood

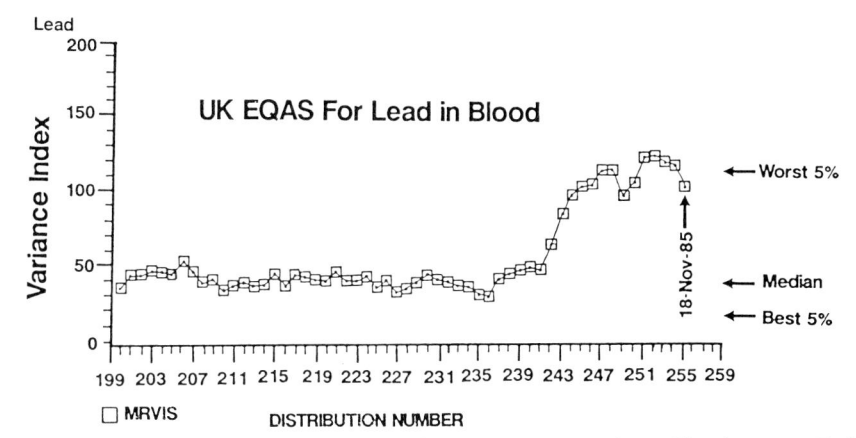

[Chart showing Variance Index vs Distribution Number, with markers for Worst 5%, Median, Best 5%, and 18-Nov-85 labeled]

Figure 3 Changes in the Mean Running Variance Index Score (MRVIS) over approximately two years for a laboratory participating in the UK National External Quality Assessment Scheme for blood lead analysis (reproduced, with permission, from ref. 17).

several decades before. These schemes demonstrated in a practical way the fundamental distinctions between relative precision and relative accuracy; they also highlighted the concept of absolute accuracy, which has proved to be a great intellectual and experimental challenge.[12,16] But there is no question that the introduction of proficiency surveys for blood lead analysis has made real accuracy a desirable and achievable goal. In Britain, there has been a steady overall improvement in laboratory performance (Figure 2), since the National External Quality Assessment Scheme[17] was introduced in 1973; however, each laboratory must carefully evaluate its own performance, and take action, on a retrospective basis (Figure 3), if the scheme is to confer real benefit. Less progress has been made in this kind of way with other elements; one reason is that the statistical data base is small, simply because of the relatively small number of laboratories which offer the more specialised analyses as a regular service.

In a certain sense, the trace elements should be amongst the easiest analytes to characterise by definitive methods and by reference methods derived from them.[18] In reality, it has been difficult to build upon the pioneering work which was done at the US National Bureau of Standards on the accurate analysis of calcium and iron in serum, and of lead in blood, using stable isotope dilution mass-spectrometry. The technique is very costly, relying as it does on the methodical identification, characterisation and elimination of sources of error. Economics work against this approach, in the absence of funding from a budget as large as that of NASA!

The limited evidence gathered so far strongly suggests that if a pool biological material is analysed for a trace element by a large network of laboratories using a variety of methods, then the consensus value for concentration is a reasonable approximation to the accurate value. Provided that the pool is large enough, that the vial-to-vial inhomogeneity is small, and that temporal stability is good, then the pool can serve as a reference material to transfer accuracy over space and time. This can be achieved by using the material either to establish the bias of a candidate reference method, e.g. with calcium in serum,[19] or to assign a concentration value to a new pool, e.g. with lead in blood haemolysate.[20]

4 CONCLUDING REMARKS

The big question is whether there will be any new incentive for clinical laboratories to use these reference materials or methods, so as to improve performance, or will we continue to rely on quality assurance which is heavily based on retrospective profiency testing? Will the trends towards laboratory accreditation and Good Laboratory Practice have an indirect impact? What will be the effect of the single market in Europe from 1992: will there be more rigorous surveillance of national or international legislation to control environmental pollution or occupational exposure to toxic elements? Will there be a big break-through involving one of the toxic elements in clinical nutrition, oncology, neurology or some other important branch of medicine that specially captures the public imagination? Each of these factors could have a bearing on laboratory workloads and quality assurance procedures, by increasing them, or by making them more complex or difficult to manage. On the other hand, what would be the effect of a revolutionary new technique, having great sensitivity, specificity, precision and accuracy, which took trace element analysis out of the laboratory into the doctor's office, the pharmacist's store, or even the patient's home? All of these places already have powerful enough microcomputers to do the necessary statistics and pattern recognition. If indeed the new technique were non-invasive, like hair analysis, it would be a certain winner!

REFERENCES

1. M.L. Kenney, Clin. Chem., 1987, 33, 328.
2. J.K. Taylor 'Quality Assurance of Chemical Measurements', Lewis Publishers Inc., Chelsea, 1987.
3. R.N. Barnett, Med. Instrumentation, 1974, 8, 14.
4. R.A. Braithwaite, These Proceedings, p.95
5. P.C. Elwood, Brit. Med. J., 1983, 286, 1553.
6. R.A. Braithwaite and S.S. Brown, Human Toxicol., 1988, 7, 503.

7. R.C. Browne, R.W. Ellis and D. Weightman, Lancet, 1974, ii, 1112, 1569.
8. J. Versieck and R. Cornelis, 'Trace Elements in Human Plasma or Serum', CRC Press Inc., Boca Raton, 1989.
9. E. Nieboer and A.A. Jusys in 'Chemical Toxicology and Clinical Chemistry of Metals' (Eds. S.S. Brown and J. Savory), Academic Press, London, 1983, p.3.
10. J. Versieck, L. Vanballenberghe, A. De Kesel, J. Hoste, B. Wallaeys, J. Vandenhaute, N. Baeck, H. Steyaert, A.R. Byrne and F.W. Sunderman Jr., Anal. Chim. Acta, 1988, 204, 63.
11. R. Gräsbeck and T. Alström (Eds.) 'Reference Values in Laboratory Medicine', John Wiley & Sons, Chichester, 1981.
12. J.P. Cali, Clin. Chem., 1973, 19, 291.
13. G.A. Uriano and C.C. Gravatt, CRC Critical Rev. Anal. Chem., 1977, 6, 361.
14. B. Welz, M.S. Wolynetz and M. Verlinden, Pure Appl. Chem., 1987, 59, 927.
15. H.A. McKenzie and L.E. Smythe (Eds.), 'Quantitative Trace Analysis of Biological Materials', Elsevier Science Publishers, Amsterdam, 1988.
16. S.S. Brown in 'Quality Control in Clinical Chemistry' (Eds. G. Anido, E.J. van Kampen, S.B. Rosalki and M. Rubin), Walter de Gruyter, Berlin, 1975, p. 417.
17. D.G. Bullock, N.J. Smith and T.P. Whitehead, Clin. Chem., 1986, 32, 1884.
18. J.H. Boutwell (Ed.), 'A National Understanding for the Development of Reference Materials and Methods for Clinical Chemistry', American Association for Clinical Chemistry, Washington, 1978.
19. S.S. Brown, M.J.R. Healy and M. Kearns, J. Clin. Chem. Clin. Biochem., 1981, 19, 395, 413.
20. R.A. Braithwaite and A.J. Girling, Fresenius Z. Anal. Chem., 1988, 332, 704.

Exposure and Exposure Assessment

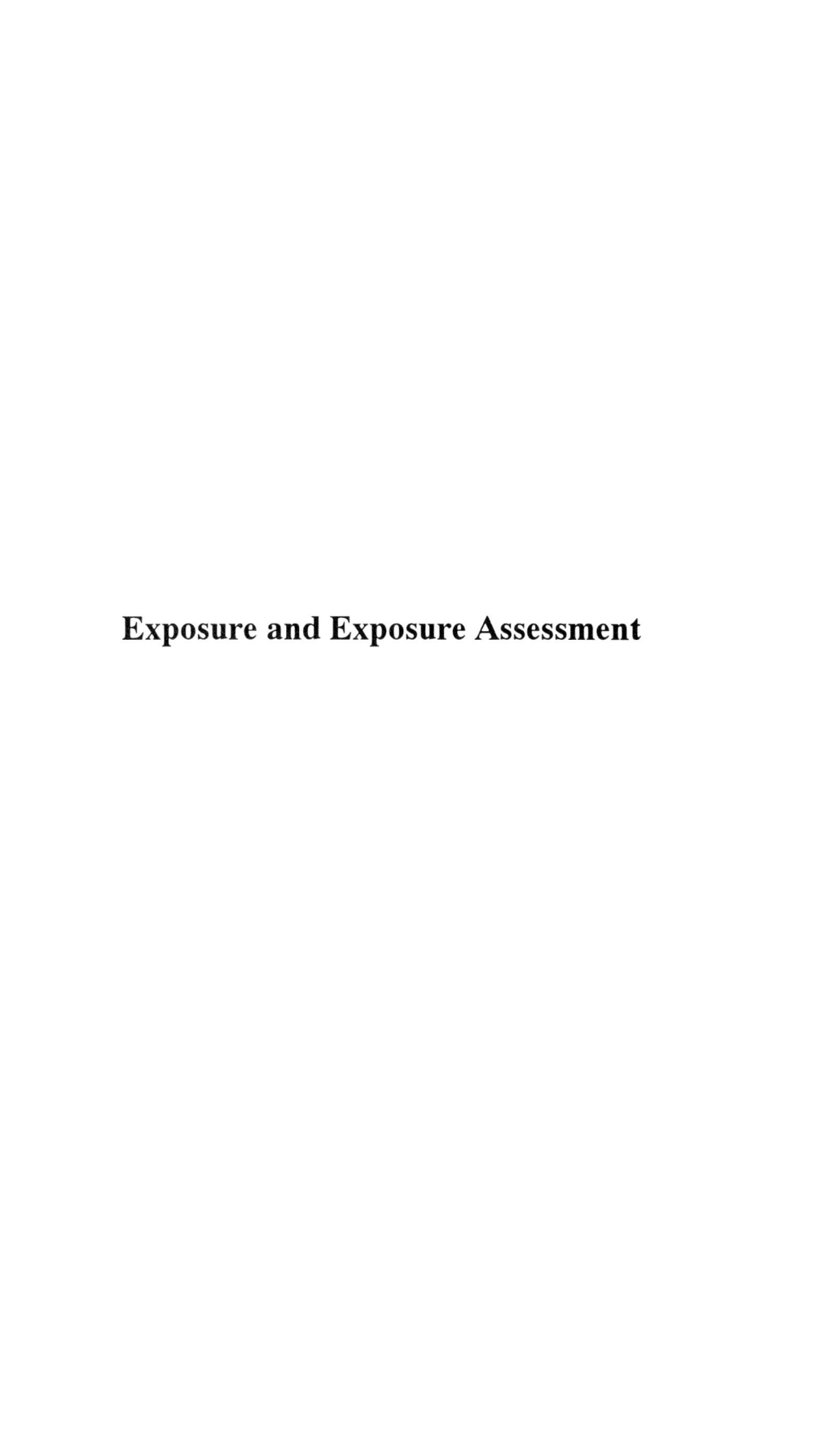

Selenium in Tap Water and Natural Water Ecosystems in Finland

Dacheng Wang, Georg Alfthan, Antti Aro, Lea Kauppi, and Jouko Soveri

NATIONAL PUBLIC HEALTH INSTITUTE, SF-003300 HELSINKI AND NATIONAL BOARD OF WATERS AND ENVIRONMENT, SF-00100 HELSINKI, FINLAND

1 INTRODUCTION

Since 1985, sodium selenate has been added to fertilizers and used nationwide in Finland[1]. Annually about 23 tons of selenium is added to the environment[2]. Upon leaching into natural waters even a small increase in selenium concentration may enhance eutrofication and at levels of a few µg/L can be toxic for some protozoa[3]. The analytical methods for selenium applied so far to waters have not been sensitive enough to detect selenium levels below 1 µg/L.

The aim of this study was to develop a sensitive method for the analysis of selenium from water samples, to assess selenium levels in different types of drinking water and natural water ecosystems and to estimate the effect of agricultural selenium fertilization and industrial pollution on environmental selenium. This paper presents the first data on the selenium concentrations in Finnish waters.

2 SAMPLE COLLECTION

New one-liter PVC bottles with PVC caps were filled with 5% nitric acid and allowed to soak for 72 h. The bottles were rinsed 6 times with distilled deionized water, and filled with distilled deionized water. After 24 h, the bottles were emptied and air-dried.

<u>Tap water</u>. Water was run for 2 minutes, the bottle washed twice with the tap water and filled.

<u>Snow</u>. New snow precipitated on 12-13th of March, 1990, was collected into a 30x45 cm plastic bag, and melted at room temperature. Samples were filtered through filter paper (Rundfilter MN 617) into one-liter PVC plastic bottles.

Infiltration water. Infiltration water was collected by Lysimeter from soils at a depth of 1.7 m, from 41 groundwater stations of the National Board of Waters and Environment. The water was then transferred into a one-liter PVC bottle, and 2.5 mL concentrated nitric acid (Merck 441, 65%) was added.

Lake, river and brook water. Water samples were taken directly into one-liter PVC bottles.
All water samples were stored at 4°C before analysis.

3   WATER SELENIUM DETERMINATION

The total selenium concentration of waters was analyzed by a modification of the fluorimetric method for tissues and biological fluids[4]. Nitric acid (0.5 mL) and a few antibumping granules were added to a 200 mL water sample in a 250 mL beaker, and then evaporated on an electric plate, until 2-3 mL was left. The remainder was transferred into glass test tubes, and 0.5 mL nitric acid, 0.5 mL $HClO_4$ and 2 drops of H_2SO_4 were added. The tubes were placed in an 110°C Al-bath overnight. The temperature was increased to 150°C for 1 hour and to 180°C for 1 hour. Then 4 drops of H_2O_2 were added after cooling, and the tubes were heated at 150°C for 10 minutes.

To reduce all selenium to selenite, 0.8 mL HCl was added and the mixture was heated for 10 minutes at 110°C. After cooling, 0.5 mL of 0.2 mol/L Na_2-EDTA, 0.5 mL of 1% hydroxylamine-HCl, and about 1 mL of NH_4OH were added to the test tubes, and the pH was adjusted to 1.5-2.0 with 4 mol/L HCl or NH_4OH. Then 0.5 mL of 0.1% 2,3-diamino-naphthalene was added, the tubes were placed in a 50°C covered water bath for 20 minutes, and then cooled in a cold water bath. Finally, 2.5 mL cyclohexane was added, the tubes were capped with a glass stopper and extracted manually for 1 minute.

Table 1   Recovery of Se (Na_2SeO_3) added to 200 mL tap water*

Se added (ng)	0	5	10	15
Se found (ng)	9.0	13.9	18.9	23.7
Recovery (%)	-	99.3	99.5	98.8
Recovery, range (%)[#]		97.3-102.5		
Mean recovery (%)	99.5			

*Mean of 4 replicates
[#]n=12

The fluorescence was measured with a Perkin-Elmer LS-5 Fluorescence Spectrometer within 2 h, at an excitation wavelength of 370 nm and an emission wavelength of 518 nm, with a slit width of 10 nm. Two blanks and a standard series of 5, 10, 15, 20, 25 and 30 ng selenium (as Na_2SeO_3) were run through all procedures with test samples.

The recovery of selenium added to 200 mL tap water was 97.3-102.5% (n=12), with an average of 99.5% (Table 1). The detection limit of the method was 1.3 ng selenium (blank+2SD), or 6.5 ng/L in a water sample.

4 RESULTS AND DISCUSSION

Selenium in Tap Water

Tap water collected from 21 cities and towns between 13th and 30th April, 1990 showed a wide range of selenium concentrations, from 13.2 ng/L in a small town to 1103 ng/L in a medium-sized industrial city (Table 2). In all analyzed tap water samples the total selenium concentration was below the recommended upper limit for drinking water in Finland of 10 µg/L. The same limit has been set also by WHO, USA and the EEC countries[5,6].

Table 2 Selenium concentration in tap water in Finland

	Location	Population	Se (ng/L)	No.	Location	Population	Se (ng/L)
1.	Central	42,500	1103	11.	Central	11,600	20.6
2.	Central	19,900	874	12.	Central	4,600	13.2
3.	Central	5,500	290	13.	S.coast	164,600	45.2
4.	Central	39,200	233	14.	S.coast	490,000	42.9
5.	Central	24,700	200	15.	S.coast	57,700	22.2
6.	Central	170,500	50.0	16.	SW.coast	160,500	52.7
7.	Central	15,900	43.4	17.	W.coast	77,400	122
8.	Central	26,800	25.6	18.	W.coast	53,700	20.9
9.	Central	14,300	25.5	19.	East	6,400	182
10.	Central	11,500	20.7	20.	East	8,300	67.1
				21.	East	34,600	55.4

In two thirds of the samples from cities and towns the selenium in tap water was lower than 100 ng/L. This level is relatively low compared with most other countries. In Greece, selenium in 256 tap water samples from 64 county towns and cities was mainly in the narrow range of 100-200 ng/L, and in only five county towns was the selenium concentration lower than 100 ng/L[7]. There was no seasonal variation of selenium concentration in Helsinki tap water. From October 17, 1989 to April 17, 1990, the tap water selenium level varied between 39.5 to 45.4 ng/L. It made Helsinki the lowest in tap water selenium concentration, compared with Antwerp, 320 ng/L and Brussels, 340-375 ng/L in Belgium; Darmstadt, 120 ng/L and 1100 ng/L and Stuttgart, 1600 ng/L in Germany;

Jerusalem, 440 ng/L in Israel; Moscow, 125 ng/L in the U.S.S.R. and Stockholm, 61 ng/L in Sweden[8].

Table 3 The effect of the purification process on tap water selenium concentration

Location	Raw water selenium (ng/L)	Tap water selenium (ng/L)
1. Turku	89.3	52.7
2. Pori	81.9	121
3. Vammala	81.7	43.4
4. Lappajärvi	65.7	13.2
5. Leppävirta	61.2	20.7
6. Kotka	59.5	22.2
7. Seinäjoki	59.2	25.6
8. Vaasa	52.9	20.9
9. Pieksämäki	41.5	25.5

Tap water selenium was decreased by the raw water purification process (Table 3). In Finland, every city and town has its own water purification system. The chemicals used were $Ca(OH)_2$, CO_2, $KMnO_4$, Flokia 20, Cl_2, NaOH, $Al(OH)_3$, NH_4Cl, $FeCl_3$, $Fe_2(SO_4)_3$, activated charcoal powder, $(C_6H_{10}O_5)_n$, $Al_2(SO_4)_3$, Na_2CO_3 etc. The decrease in selenium by the purification process may be due to selenite binding tightly to iron and aluminium oxides[9], which are then precipitated.

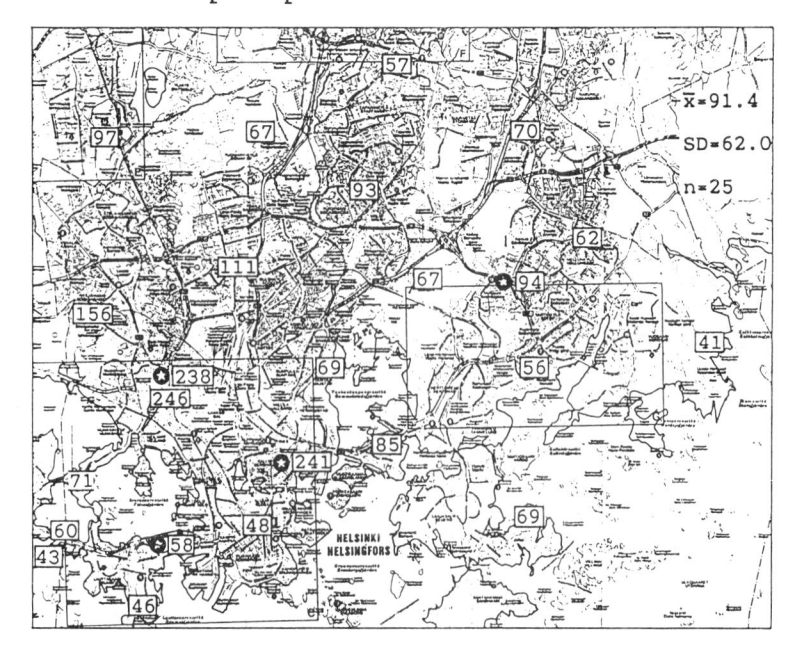

Fig.1 Selenium in snow in the Helsinki area (ng/l)

○ power plant

Selenium in Snow

The mean selenium concentration of 25 snow samples collected in the Helsinki area on 8-9th of March, 1990, from the same precipitation, was 91.4 ng/L, range 41.8-246 ng/L (Fig 1). In 20 samples the selenium concentration was lower than 100 ng/L. Two samples out of four collected in the vicinity of electric power plants had selenium concentration higher than 100 ng/L (241 and 238 ng/L). This may be due to coal or oil burning release. Samples far from the city centre had lower selenium concentrations. The selenium concentration in snow samples collected from groundwater stations of the National Board of Waters and Environment in the countryside between 15th February and 9th April, 1990 were low in selenium, with an average of 28.7 ng/L. It seems that urbanization increases atmospheric selenium.

Selenium concentration in snow in Antwerp, Belgium was 290 ng/L[8]; in Yokohama, Japan 33 ng/L on March 8th,1987; in Tokyo, 44 ng/L on January 5th and 132 ng/L on February 2nd, 1987[10]. Because there are large differences in the selenium concentration of snow within cities, the significance of results from single samples is doubtful.

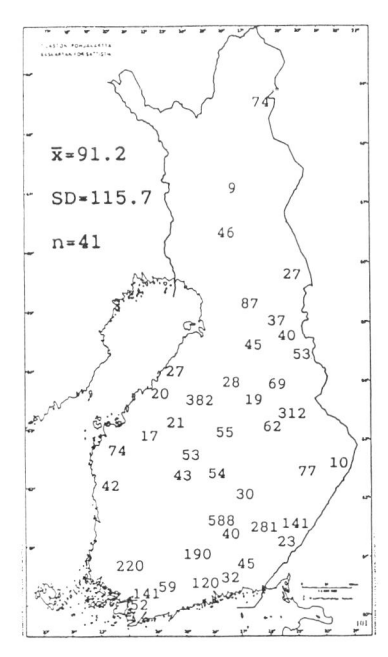

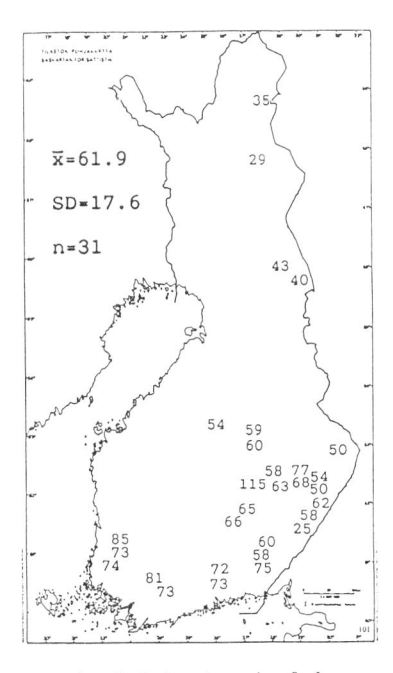

Fig.2 Selenium in infiltration water (ng/l)

Fig.3 Selenium in lake water (ng/l)

Selenium in Infiltration Water

Infiltration means the penetration of meltwater or rainwater from the soil surface into the soil. The infiltration water flows through the soil under the action of gravity as percolation water. The groundwater observation stations of the National Board of Waters and Environment are background stations in nearly natural surroundings, located in areas where the groundwater quality has not been appreciably affected by local environmental disturbances[11]. The infiltration water samples in this study were collected by Lysimeter at a depth of 1.7 m, representing different types of soils.

The total selenium concentration in infiltration water varied widely, ranging from 9 to 588 ng/L (Fig 2). All 9 high-selenium samples (higher than 100 ng/L) out of 41 were south of the 64° northern latitude where most of the country's population are living. There was no significant relationship between snow selenium and infiltration water selenium (n=19). Neither were there any significant associations between the selenium concentration of infiltration water and type of soil. So, the high selenium concentrations in some infiltration water samples may just depend on the selenium concentration of the bed rock.

Selenium in Lake Water

Water samples from 31 lakes were collected between the 22nd of March and the 26th of April, 1990. Of the lakes, 13 were surrounded by cultivated fields, considered as agriculturally affected areas; 18 lakes from areas not affected by agriculture were selected as controls.

The average total selenium concentration in these 31 lakes was 61.9 ng/L (SD 17.6)(Fig 3). The range of selenium was rather narrow, 25-115 ng/L, less than five fold. There was no significant difference in total selenium between agriculturally affected and non-affected lakes. In samples from the 4 lakes located north of the 64° northern latitude the selenium concentration was significantly lower (mean=36.6 ng/L) than in the other lakes in the south (65.6 ng/L).

Table 4 Selenium in river and brook water

Location	No.	Mean Selenium (ng/L)	SD
Central	4	110	17.7
Southern coast	13	89.7	19.5
Western coast	4	55.5	5.0

In Norway, selenium in water samples from 40 lakes distributed throughout the country was 135 ng/L[12]. The Great Lakes in North America had selenium concentrations ranging from 71 to 3000 ng/L during 1980-1985[13]. In the Netherlands, Yssel lake selenium was 1850 ng/L[8]. Thus the selenium concentration in Finnish lakes was relatively low.

Selenium in Rivers and Brooks

River water samples were taken in April, 1990. The selenium concentration in these rivers differed between the central, southern coast and western coast areas (Table 4). To find out the reasons for the differences more samples will be needed.

Table 5 Seasonal variation of selenium in river water (ng/L)

Location	Date	Selenium	Location	Date	Selenium
Läyliäinen	21.2.90	145	Voutila	26.2.90	221
	1.4.90	118		24.3.90	170
Tolkinkylä	26.2.90	148	Östersundom	26.2.90	66.9
	16.4.90	90.5		13.4.90	52.5
Vantaa	26.2.90	134	Husö	24.3.90	91.6
	16.4.90	101		15.4.90	71.4

Compared with the samples taken in the same places earlier, the river water selenium concentration decreased from February to March and April (Table 5). This decrease may be caused by the melting of snow which may dissolve some selenium from soils and transfer it to the rivers.

There are few data on river water selenium from other countries. In the greater Tokyo area of Japan, 23 samples from 4 rivers had a mean selenium of 110 ng/L, ranging between 20-630 ng/L[14]. In Norway, two rivers Lora and Skjoma had selenium concentrations of 120 and 80 ng/L, respectively[12].

5 SUMMARY

The total selenium concentration of tap water, snow, infiltration water, lake and river water was studied in different areas of Finland. Water samples were preconcentrated by evaporating and the selenium concentration analysed fluorometrically after wet digestion. The recovery of selenium from 200 mL tap water was on average 99.5% with a detection limit of 1.3 ng selenium (blank+2SD) or 6.5 ng/L selenium in a water sample. The method can be used to determine selenium in tap water and natural water samples. The total tap water selenium concentration in 21 Finnish cities and towns was lower than the limit for drinking water. The water purification process generally decreased the selenium concentration. The mean selenium concentration in snow in the Helsinki area was higher than that in rural areas. The load of selenium in infiltration water may depend on the selenium concentration of the bedrock. There were no significant differences between the selenium concentrations of agriculturally affected and non-affected lakes. River water selenium decreased from early spring to late spring within one to two months.

In conclusion, the selenium concentration in Finnish tap water and natural water samples was relatively low compared with other countries. There is no evidence that agricultural fertilization has increased the selenium concentration of natural waters in Finland.

5 ACKNOWLEDGMENTS

This research was supported by the Maj and Tor Nessling Foundation.

6 REFERENCES

1. P.Koivistoinen and J.K.Huttunen, Annals Clin. Res., 1986, 18, 13.
2. J.E.Oldfield, Proc. Selenium-Tellurium Development Assoc., 1988.
3. E.A.Davis, K.J.Maier and A.W.Knight, California Agric., Jan.-Feb., 1988.
4. G.Alfthan, Anal. Chim. Acta, 1984, 165, 187.
5. Water Quality Criteria. Environmental Protection Agency, Washington, D.C. (EPA-R3-73-033), March, 1973.
6. Environmental Protection Agency, Drinking Water and Health. Recommendation of the National Academy of Sciences, Federal Register, 1977, 42, 35773.
7. M.S.Bratakos, Th.F.Zafiropoulos, P.A.Siskos and P.V.Ioannou, Sci. Total Environ., 1988, 76, 49.
8. H.Robberecht and R.Van Grieken, Talanta, 1982, 29, 823.
9. J.H.Howard, III., Trace Subst. in Environ. Health, V, Columbia, Missouri, University of Missouri Press, 1971, 485.
10. T.Ishikawa and Y.Hashimoto, Bunseki Kagaku, 1988, 37, 344 (in Japanese).
11. J.Soveri, Publ. Water Res. Inst. 63, National Board of Waters, Finland, 1985.
12. R.O.Allen and E.Steinnes, NGU-BULL, 1987, 409, 35.
13. R.Rossmann and J.Barres, J.Great Lakes Res., 1988, 14, 188.
14. S.Suzuki, S.Koizumi, H.Harada, K.Ito and T.Totani, Annu. Rep. Tokyo Metropol. Res. Lab. Publ. Health, 1970, 22, 153 (in Japanese).

Release of Aluminium from Coated Saucepans

Andrew Taylor
TRACE ELEMENTS LABORATORY, DEPARTMENT OF CLINICAL BIOCHEMISTRY
AND CLINICAL NUTRITION, ST. LUKE'S HOSPITAL, GUILDFORD, GU1 3NT
AND
ROBENS INSTITUTE OF HEALTH AND SAFETY, UNIVERSITY OF SURREY,
GUILDFORD, GU2 5XH, ENGLAND

1 INTRODUCTION

Aluminium cooking utensils and saucepans have been used since 1890[1] and experiments to determine whether any of the metal will dissolve from the surface and add to the load of the contents were first reported in 1892[2]. Weighed strips of aluminium metal were suspended in various media and the loss in weight determined after six days. This gravimetric approach demonstrated that greatest solubility was found with food-acids at 1-5% solution, followed by white wine, red wine, brandy, 50% alcohol and coffee. Tea and beer caused no measurable aluminium weight loss. Similar experiments by other workers examined the effects of water, acetic acid, lemonade, milk and soda[3-6]. Release of aluminium by foodstuffs was further thoroughly investigated in the laboratories of the Lancet[7]. All these experiments confirmed the loss of aluminium demonstrated by Lange and Schmid[2] and showed that release of the metal was enhanced when the contents were acidic or basic. Authors were also in agreement and concluded that the quantities dissolved were too small to be of any relevance to the health of consumers.

Investigations have been repeated in recent years with the quantitative analysis of aluminium in the contents of the cookware carried out by the sensitive technique of electrothermal atomisation atomic absorption spectrometry (ETAAS). The observations of one hundred years ago have been largely confirmed[8-10] and it has been further suggested that leaching of aluminium is promoted by fluoride at 10 ppm.[11]

The gastrointestinal absorption of aluminium is normally very poor. The normal dietary intake is approximately five mg and metabolic balance studies indicate that in healthy individuals absorption of aluminium is less than 0.1% and that any assimilated is readily excreted in the urine.[12] The absorption of insoluble aluminium compounds used to treat gastric acidity is likewise very limited although the use of these agents to limit hyperphosphataemia in patients with chronic renal failure can cause high concentrations of aluminium in serum.[13,14] Thus, there are some situations, or groups of subjects, where intestinal absorption of aluminium is greater than is usually expected. Experimental work by Slanina and his colleagues[15] demonstrated that aluminium as the citrate complex was easily absorbed across the rat intestine and, in addition, the aluminium was retained at high concentrations in many body tissues. This enhanced bioavailability was also demonstrated in recent examples of patients who were co-treated with aluminium and Shohl's solution (citric acid and sodium citrate), who developed neurological symptoms of aluminium encelopathy.[16,17] Rapid absorption may also be facilitated by changes to the intestinal mucosa with accumulation of aluminium and signs of encephalopathy[18,19]

Associations between the concentrations of aluminium in drinking water and dementia-related disease have been demonstrated although a causal link has not been established.[20,21] However, a relationship between intake of aluminium and Alzheimer's or other dementia-related diseases cannot be discounted and further work requiring accurate determination of the metal in water, food and biological samples is proceeding.

In view of the associations between aluminium and dementia there is an increasing concern among the general public.[22] Many individuals have chosen to reduce their daily aluminium intake by the use of water purifiers or of bottled mineral water. In response to public perception of aluminium, some manufacturers have produced cookware with a seal or coating to limit the release of aluminium into the contents.

This study was designed to test the effectiveness of the coatings used by different manufacturers in prevention of release of aluminium.

2 MATERIALS AND METHODS

Samples

Coated of hard-anodised aluminium saucepans of 16 - 26.6 cm diameter were obtained new from nine manufacturers. A stainless steel and an uncoated aluminium pan were also examined.

Each saucepan was washed clean, rinsed twice with deionised water and washed again by addition of deionised water, which was boiled within the pan.

Release of Aluminium from Coated Saucepans 59

Table 1. Coated aluminium cookware used to examine release of aluminium

Saucepan A   Berndes Bonanza
Saucepan B   Tefal Graphite
Saucepan C   Salt and Jukes
Saucepan D   Choice Cookware Scanpan
Saucepan E   Mellerware
Saucepan F   Russell Hobbs Tower Sovereign
Saucepan G   Meyer Circulon
Saucepan H   BMS New Premier
Saucepan I   ICTC Look

Test protocol

* 500 mL of deionised water was added to the clean saucepan and boiled for ten min
* The residual volume was measured and an aliquot taken for measurement of aluminium
* The saucepan was rinsed with tap water boiled within the pan
* 500 mL tap water was added to the clean saucepan and boiled for ten min
* The residual volume was measured and an aliquot taken for measurement of aluminium
* 225 g washed, cut rhubarb and 200 mL tap water were placed into the saucepan, cooked for ten min and weighed

Analyses

The cooked rhubarb samples were mixed in acid-washed plastic containers with cleaned plastic cutlery. Weighed aliquots were digested with nitric and perchloric acids. Residues were dissolved in dilute nitric acid and the aluminium concentrations measured by ETAAS. The NBS lyophilised reference material, bovine liver 1577a, was also digested and the aluminium measured.[23]

Nitric acid was added to water samples to give a concentration of 1% (v/v) and the concentrations of aluminium measured by ETAAS.[24] Serum-based reference materials with known concentrations were used to monitor within-batch and between-batch reproducibility and specimens of water, dialysis fluids and sera, distributed as a part of the Guildford External Quality Assessment Scheme, were analysed to measure accuracy.[25,26]

3 RESULTS

Blank values

Aluminium concentrations in the deionised water, tap water and rhubarb/water test mixture were: Deionised water, 1 µg/L, tap water, 6 µg/L, and rhubarb sample, 1.26 µg/g.

Test samples

The results were used to calculate the amounts of aluminium extracted form each pan by the cooking procedures (Table 2).

Table 2. Aluminium extracted from the saucepans by deionised water, tap water and rhubarb.

Saucepan	Deionised water µg	Tap water µg	Rhubarb µg
Stainless steel	0.6	0.50	<1
Uncoated aluminium	143.0	5923	13115
A	7.0	2.4	<1
B	2.6	0.6	<1
C	17.9	67.8	105
D	9.8	45.2	<1
E	17.8	24.5	<1
F	2.0	2.2	<1
G	1.7	2.0	62
H	33.8	578.4	146
I	4.3	2.5	<1

Very little aluminium was present in samples obtained from the stainless steel pan. These results were equivalent to the blank values and indicate that the precautions taken to prevent extraneous contamination had been successful.

The aluminium content of samples heated in the uncoated aluminium saucepan showed that leaching will readily occur and could contribute large amounts to the daily intake. The stewed rhubarb sample contained approximately 13 mg aluminium in a portion that weighed 320 g.

The coatings used on the other aluminium saucepans were generally effective. With five saucepans, only very small amounts were added to the water samples and even with the other saucepans the additions were much less than occurred with the uncoated pan. The aluminium content of rhubarb did not increase when cooked in six of the coated saucepans. The concentration increment measured in the other three samples was less than 150 µg in a portion of approximately 300 g.

4 DISCUSSION

Extraction of aluminium from the uncoated saucepan was similar to that previously demonstrated by others,[1-9] with large amounts released by acidic food. Measured dietary intake of aluminium is approximately 5 mg per day with small amounts contributed from the drinking water. Use of aluminium saucepans could cause the intake to be increased several fold, with enhancement of the concentrations in certain foods and in water or other liquids heated in these pans.

Although the bioavailability of aluminium from foods, water and other liquids has not been determined, some of the increased dietary load consequent upon cooking with aluminium saucepans could be absorbed. This would have important implications if a causal link between intake of aluminium and dementia were to be established.

This demonstration that the coatings effectively reduced or prevented aluminium release, from the saucepans into the contents, will provide some reassurance to those who are concerned about this question and wish to limit aluminum intake.

It has been suggested the fluoride in water will increase the rate at which aluminium is extracted from the metallic surface.[11] The fluoride concentration of the tap water used in this study (measured by Thames Water Authority) was 221 µg/L (0.221 ppm). This is low compared to many other areas and would have had little or no effect on loss of aluminium from the saucepans.

The results reported here were obtained with only one example of each pan and may, therefore, not be representative of the specimens examined. However, there did not appear to be any problems relating to excessive contamination and it is unlikely that the saucepans used differed greatly from other prepared by the same manufacturing process.

The saucepans tested were new. It is probable that the structure and integrity of coatings will alter with use and/or washing and that some may deteriorate more rapidly than others. As the coatings become aged it is likely that the amounts of aluminium extracted will increase.

5 CONCLUSIONS

1. Uncoated aluminium saucepans can contribute significant amounts of the metal to the food, and cooking in these could increase daily intake to several times greater than normal. Acidic foods are especially efficient at extraction of aluminium.

2. At least when new, coatings used on available saucepans are effective in reducing the extraction of aluminium.

3. The degree of reduction in extraction varies between the coatings used by different manufacturers. Some prevent any aluminium leaching but others allow a little contamination of the contents.

This study was part of an investigation carried out by the Good Housekeeping Institute and was featured in the March 1990 edition of Good Housekeeping Magazine.

6 REFERENCES

1. E.E. Smith, 'Aluminium Compounds in Food', Paul B. Hoeber, New York, 1928, p 24.
2. G. Lunge and E. Schmid, Zeitschrift Angew. chemie., 1892, p.7.
3. W. Ohlmuller and R. Heise, Arb.a.d.k. Gesundheitsamte, 1893, 8, 377.
4. Dr. Plagge and G. Lebbin, Veraff. a.d.Geb. d.Militär-Sanitätswes., 1893, 3, 1.
5. M. Mansfeld, Zschrf Unters. Nahrungs- u.Genussmitt., 1904, 8, 765.
6. F. von Fillinger, Zschrf Unters. Nahrungs-u.Genussmitt. 1908, 16, 232.
7. Editorial, Lancet, an 4 1913, p 54.
8. J. Savory, J.R. Nicholsson and M.R. Wills, Nature, 1987, 327, 107.
9. T. Inoue, H. Ishiwata, Y. Kunitoshi, J. Agric. Food Chem., 1988, 36, 599.
10. K.Tennakone and S. Wickramanayake, Nature, 1987, 325, 202.
11. K.Tennakone and S. Wickramanayake, Nature, 1987, 325, 398.
12. J.L. Greger and M.J. Baier, Fd. Chem. Toxicol., 1983, 21, 473.
13. W.D. Kaehney, A.P. Hegg and A.C. Alfrey, New Engl. J. Med., 1977, 296, 1389.
14. S.P. Andreoli, J.M. Bergstein and D.J. Sherrard, New Emgl. J. Med., 1984, 310, 1079.
15. P. Slanina, Y. Falkeborn, Y. Frech and A. Cedergren, Fd. Chem. Toxicol., 1984, 22, 391.
16. A.A. Bakir, D.O. Hhyhorczuk, S. Ahmed, S.M. Hessl, P.S. Levy, R. Spemgler and G. Dunea, Clin. Nephrol., 1989, 31, 40.
17. B.B. Kirschbaum and A.C. Schoolwerth, Am. J. Med. Sci., 1989, 296, 9.
18. J.M. Campistol, A. Cases, A. Botey and A. Revert, Nephron, 1989, 51, 103.
19. D.J. Withers, A.S. Woolf, J.C. Kingswood, W.N. Tsang and M.A. Mansell, Lancet, 1989, ii, 674.

20. D.P. Perl, D.C. Gajdusek, R.M. Garruto, R.T. Yanagihara and C.J. Gibbs Jr, Science, 1982, 217, 1053.
21. C.N. Martyn, C. Osmond, J.A. Edwardsson, D.J.P. Barker, E.C. Harris and R.F. Lacey, Lancet, 1989, i, 59.
22. Anon. Aluminium. In 'Which?' consumers Association, London, June 1990, p 351.
23. R. Hughes and A. Taylor, In 'Aluminium and Other Trace Elements in Renal Disease', ed A. Taylor, Bailliere Tindall, Eastbouorne, 1986, p 303.
24. B.J. Starkey, A. Taylor and A.W. Walker, in 'Aluminium and Other Trace Elements in Renal Disease', ed A. Taylor, Bailliere Tindall, Eastbourne, 1986, p 177.
25. A. Taylor, Fresenius Z. Anal. Chem., 1988, 332, 616.
26. A. Taylor and R.J. Briggs, J. Anal. Atomic Spectrom., 1986, 1, 391.

Constraints in Biological Monitoring

P. Grandjean

INSTITUTE OF COMMUNITY HEALTH, ODENSE UNIVERSITY, DK-5000 ODENSE, DENMARK

1 INTRODUCTION

Emphasis in toxicology is shifting toward long-term exposures to toxic chemicals and their chronic, delayed or subclinical effects. This trend is an obvious result of the improved prevention of acute poisoning. Moreover, a need for increased awareness concerning chronic exposures is based on the conjecture that such exposures may play a role in causation of diseases with a multifactorial etiology. Methods used in biological monitoring must face the challenges that these developments represent.

2 INACCESSIBLE COMPARTMENTS

Biological monitoring necessitates repeated sampling and analysis of human tissue and body fluids for analysis. Certain restrictions apply with regard to the type of methods acceptable for such routine examinations of healthy individuals. Thus, most frequently biological monitoring is based on chemical analysis of blood samples. However, the trace element concentration in blood may not necessarily reflect the levels in target tissues or body depots.

With lead, the target tissue is the central nervous system, particularly in children. The half-time of lead in this compartment in humans is unknown, but it must be considerably longer than that in blood. Thus, the lead concentration in blood is unlikely to represent the amount of lead that has reached the sensitive nervous tissue. For biological monitoring purposes, the nervous system is an inaccessible compartment.

Other approaches have been attempted, *e.g.* by analysing lead in mineralized tissues, such as teeth. In these storage depots, lead has a long half-time that may not be much different from that in the nervous system. We conducted a study of a cohort of children in the municipality of Århus, Denmark. Among those children that attended the first school class, 1302 donated one or more deciduous teeth for lead analysis. Detailed examination was then carried out of a nested case-control group identified on the basis of the lead concentration in the circumpulpal dentin. The "case" group with concentrations above 0.090 µmol/g was matched to control children among those with concentrations below 0.024 µmol/g; matching was performed for gender and parental socioeconomic status. The lead levels in dentin indicated considerable differences in lead exposures during the active life of the tissue, i.e. from the time of tooth eruption to the shedding about six years later. During this time interval, the developing nervous system is believed to be very sensitive to toxic exposures.

At the age of 9 years, a blood sample was collected for lead analysis. The children with the lowest dentin levels (N=76) had low blood-lead (B-Pb) concentrations of 0.08-0.70 µmol/L and a geometric mean of 0.18 µmol/L. In comparison, the children with the highest dentin lead levels (N=70), had B-Pbs of 0.08-0.63 µmol/L and a geometric mean of 0.28 µmol/L.[1] Thus, B-Pb was significantly

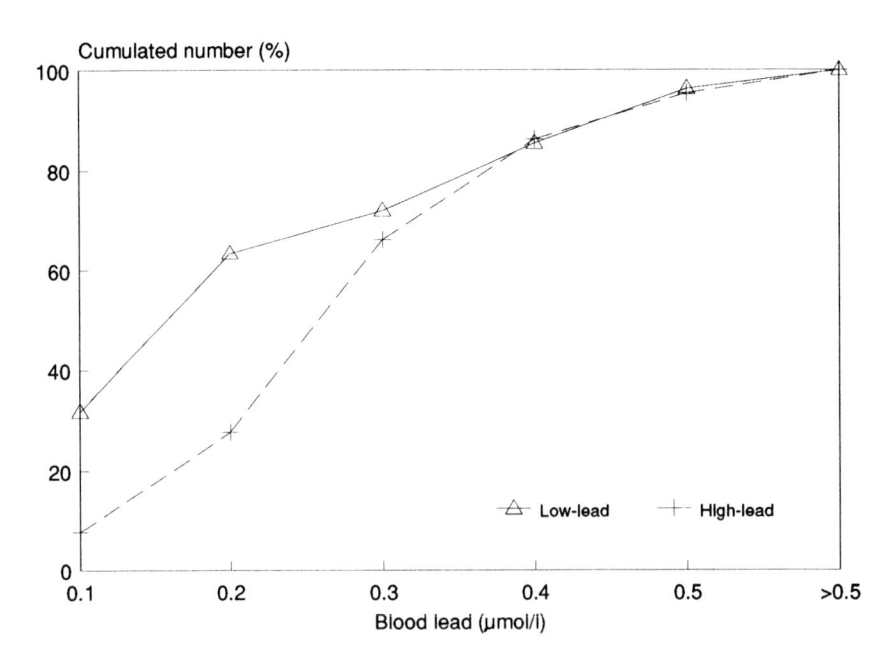

Fig. 1 Distribution of blood-lead concentrations in two groups of children with low and high lead levels stored in their deciduous teeth

higher in the high tooth-lead group than in the low-level group. As shown in Fig. 1, this difference is due to the fact that most of the children with low lead concentrations in their teeth also had a B-Pb below 0.2 µmol/L.

Further, the current lead status, as indicated by the B-Pb level, was poorly correlated with the cumulated past exposure, as assessed by the dentine lead level. A close relationship between these two measures would not be anticipated, unless lead absorption and retention were fairly constant. This experience has emphasized that trace element concentrations in superficial compartments must be interpreted cautiously.

4 AMBIGUOUS REFERENCE LEVELS

Biological monitoring data are only meaningful if they can be compared, either within the same individual over time or with appropriate reference levels. With some trace elements, the reference intervals have decreased considerably during recent years. In the case of lead, this decrease in many countries is due to a fortunate reduction of environmental pollution. However, this decrease may not necessarily be sufficient to eliminate chronic toxicity.

The Århus children with the highest lead exposures showed significantly depressed test results when compared to the control group, and a detailed analysis of potential confounders showed that lead played an important role.[2] This finding is disconcerting, because the B-Pb levels were mostly below 0.5 µmol/L (10 µg/100 mL),[1] a level that is usually considered safe. Although neurobehavioural lead toxicity in this low exposure range cannot yet be considered proven beyond doubt, our findings along with data from other countries raise serious questions concerning the safety of current environmental lead exposures.

Trace elements have always occurred in the biosphere, and a certain level of exposure is an inevitable part of natural life on this planet. However, the magnitude of human exposure to these substances today may differ considerably from those in which our genetic material developed by means of natural selection. As originally suggested by Patterson,[3] only a small fraction of modern lead exposures is of natural origin. Following this line of reasoning, reference levels based on natural exposures may be very low.

We have examined this possibility with regard to lead and cadmium, two trace elements that both occur in mineralised tissues (Fig. 2). Thus, in premolars from up to 5000-year old remains of Nubians and from 500-year old mummies of Inuits from Greenland, the lead concentrations were very low; modern teeth contained 10-100 times more lead. In contrast, cadmium concentrations varied by 30-fold in the two prehistorical populations, and modern-day cadmium levels were in the lower range of this interval.[4] In connection with Patterson's data, these findings suggest that the impact of current environmental cadmium pollution is limited when compared to the considerable consequences of lead pollution. Again, this evidence adds to the concerns regarding the safety of current environmental lead exposures.

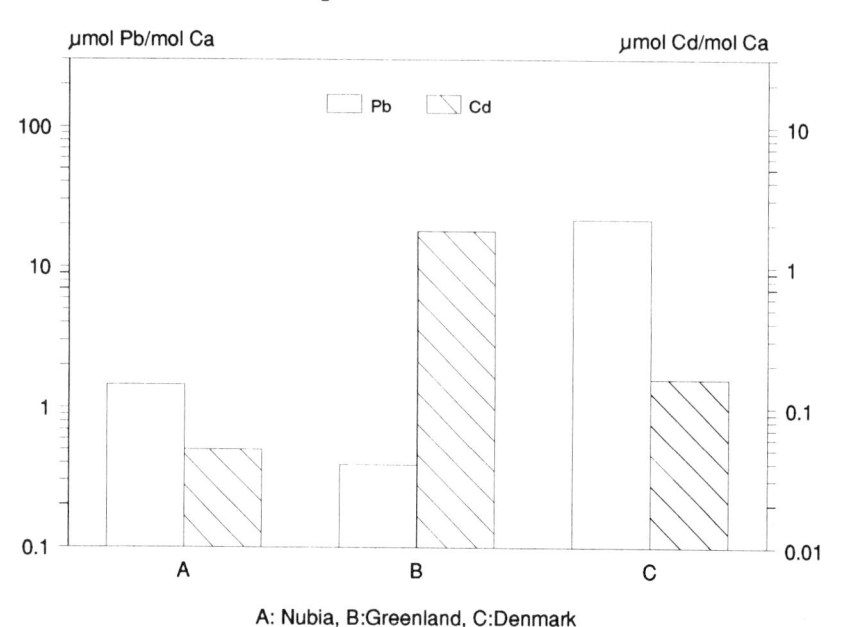

Fig. 2 Average concentrations of lead (scale on the left) and cadmium (scale on the right) in circumpulpal dentin from A: nine ancient Nubians (5300-3300 b.p.), B: three Inuit mummies (500 b.p.) and C: thirty-three current-day Danes.

5 NONSPECIFIC EFFECTS

A recent review of the scientific literature on clinical intoxications[5] showed that 220 environmental chemicals (drugs and natural toxins excluded) had caused documented systemic toxicity in humans. This number is perhaps surprisingly low, in particular when compared to the thousands of chemicals known to cause adverse effects in experimental animals. However, not all cases of human poisoning may be reported in the literature, and the information published is frequently too incomplete to allow a critical judgment concerning the chemical etiology of the clinical effects. Cases without a clear-cut causal relation were obviously left out of consideration in the survey. Thus, when the exposure has been mixed, or, as in some patients, a particular disposition or pre-existing disease may have exacerbated the clinical picture, these cases were disregarded. Despite these shortcomings, this database is of interest when evaluating the specificity of toxic effects in humans.

Most of the individual clinical effects seen in cases of intoxication had a very low specificity, i.e., they could be caused by a large number of compounds. This observation is perhaps not surprising when considering that the number of pathological reactions within the human body must be limited and that every individual chemical cannot be expected to cause a specific effect. However, the virtual absence of specific effects certainly complicates the search for etiologic diagnoses. In addition, this situation will complicate the recognition of early stages of a chronic intoxication, because the nonspecific effects will be even more difficult to determine when they develop insidiously. Trace elements are no different in this regard than other toxic substances. This problem adds further to the difficulty in determining the upper safe exposure levels, as reflected in biological monitoring results.

6 SIGNIFICANCE OF RESERVE CAPACITY

The human body has a certain capacity to withstand potentially adverse effects of environmental exposures. Thus, exposures to trace elements and other toxic substances may not necessarily result in obvious toxicity, specific or non-specific; low doses could conceivably cause a weakening of the body defenses, i.e. a decrease in reserve capacity. This effect may not be readily observable, but it could lead to increased susceptibility to subsequent exposures to other hazards.

To examine the possible significance of this factor, we examined the blood regeneration following phlebotomy (0.45 L) in 25 men with occupational lead exposure as compared to a control group of 25 other industrial workers.[6] Blood lead levels in the exposed group averaged 2.14 µmol/L (44 µg/100 mL). On day 15, the lead workers showed a significant delay in blood regeneration, as demonstrated by lower hemoglobin concentration, and erythrocyte and reticulocyte counts. Despite normal hematological findings in the initial examination of the lead-exposed workers, the lead exposure caused a decreased reserve capacity for blood formation. The important conclusion is that this effect became prominent only after blood loss by phlebotomy that unmasked the decreased rate of blood regeneration in the lead-exposed workers.

Physiological information and a small number of clinical studies suggest that reserve capacity could be a useful notion in other situations. Thus, recent studies have suggested that certain degenerative neurological diseases, such as parkinsonism and amyotrophic lateral sclerosis, may be due to accumulated effects of age and environmentally-induced damages.[7] Thus, early neurotoxic effects can be looked upon as a decrease in reserve capacity. No ill-health will be apparent in association with the exposure, but the decreased reserve capacity will limit the ability to compensate for age-related decrements. Thus, normal cell attrition and, perhaps, cumulation of other adverse influences may subsequently unmask the dysfunctions many years later (Fig. 3). The absence of an adverse effect in association with a current or recent exposure may therefore not be a guarantee that the exposure has been innocuous.

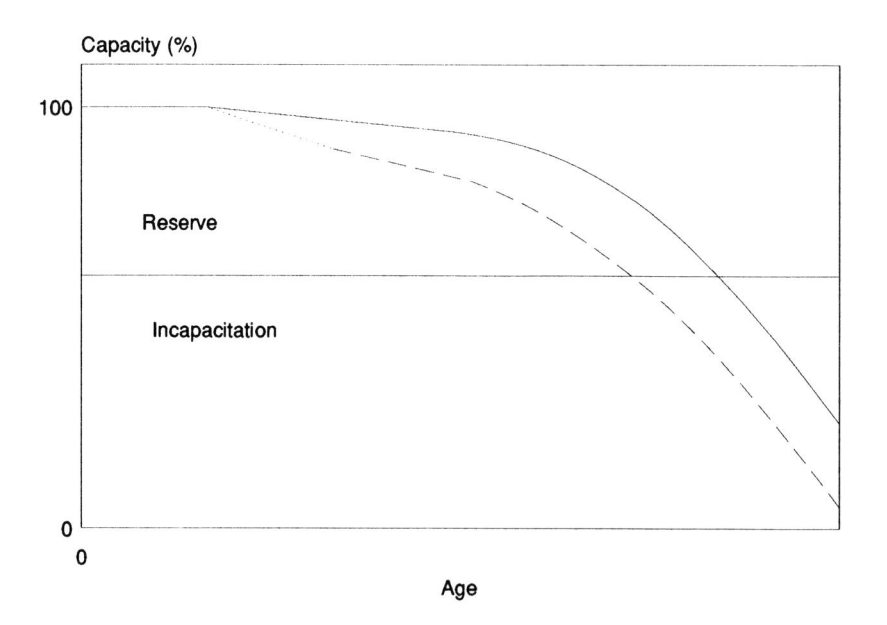

Fig. 3 With age, the capacity of various organ functions tends to decrease, but clinical symptoms may not appear until no reserve capacity is left and the threshold for incapacitation is reached. However, a toxic exposure, e.g. in young adulthood, may eliminate some of the reserve capacity (dotted line), and the subsequent age-dependent loss of functional capacity (dashed line) then results in clinical symptoms many years later, but much before such symptoms would otherwise have developed.

Evidence from studies of kidney function also suggest that a reserve capacity exists in this organ.[8] For example, a major part of the nephrons must be lost before any changes can be seen in serum creatinine. Further, glomerular blood flow and creatinine clearance will normally increase in response to a high-protein meal. However, this response is absent in patients with limited kidney function, probably because the glomerular blood flow is already at its maximum. Nephrotoxic trace elements may well affect this reserve capacity, thereby rendering the kidneys more susceptible to subsequent damage.

The notion of reserve capacity may also be useful in a wider sense. The lungs can in a physiological sense have a certain reserve function, as seen in connection with the development of chronic bronchitis.[9] Further, the metabolism of many chemicals in the body can be restricted by, e.g., enzyme inhibition or decreased availability of glutathione. Thus, biochemically, reserve capacity may also be a useful term, and trace elements may become important models for research in this area.

7 INDIVIDUAL SUSCEPTIBILITY

The existence of some forms of reserve capacity will obviously result in different degrees of individual susceptibility in human populations. Thus, if trace element exposures have tapped the reserves without causing frank disease, the individuals concerned will be in severe trouble when they meet their next exposure.

The existence of many types of genetic predisposition to toxic effects of chemicals is well documented.[10] As an extreme example, Wilson's disease causes profound genetic predisposition to exposure to copper. The associated liver damage can be decreased by early detection of the disease and subsequent treatment with low-copper diet.

Genetic polymorphisms are known for numerous enzymes that metabolize foreign compounds, and interindividual differences in enzymatic activity can explain certain cases of hypersusceptibility to drugs and other chemicals. Although the implications of these observations are unclear at present, they tend to support the notion that inherited factors may be involved in individual predisposition to toxic effects of environmental chemicals, including trace elements.

In clinical practice and in epidemiology, the same exposure may lead to vastly different effects in different individuals. In the past, we have referred to "individual susceptibility" when describing such events without any exhaustive understanding of the mechanisms involved. However, with the improved knowledge of the environmental and genetic factors behind such vulnerability, we need to clarify these mechanisms to be able to offer better protection of the hyper-susceptible individuals.

8 CHALLENGES FOR FUTURE RESEARCH

Biological monitoring has proven tremendously useful in many situations, and these techniques have without doubt resulted in great preventive benefits. However, as more information becomes available, several shortcomings appear.

A major problem is due to the kinetic behaviour of trace elements that results in varying degrees of organ retention. A simple analysis of a blood sample may convey much useful information, but it rarely allows any detailed evaluation with regard to the amounts of the trace element that have reached the target organ.

Under most exposure circumstances, trace elements constitute only part of the etiological panorama. As a parallel, many diseases have now been shown to be of multifactorial origin. Thus, a variety of factors can influence the course and severity of a disease. An important obstacle in determining the significance of trace element exposures in this regard is the non-specificity of most of the adverse effects. Also, increased individual susceptibility of whatever cause is likely to influence the dose-effect or dose-response relationships. Due to these considerations, reserve capacity may be a notion of wide significance.

9 REFERENCES

1. O.N. Hansen, A. Trillingsgaard, I. Beese, T. Lyngbye and P. Grandjean, Neurotoxicol.Behav.Teratol., 1989, 11, 205.
2. T. Lyngbye, P. Grandjean, O. Nørby Hansen, P.J. Jørgensen, Scand. J. Clin. Lab. Invest., 1990 (in press).
3. C.C. Patterson, Arch.Environ.Health, 1965, 11, 344.
4. P. Grandjean and P.J. Jørgensen, Environ.Res., in press.
5. R.D. Kimbrough, K.R. Mahaffey, P. Grandjean, S.H. Sandø and D.D. Ruttstein, 'Clinical Effects of Environmental Chemicals: A Guide to Etiologic Diagnosis', Hemisphere, New York, 1989.
6. P. Grandjean, B.M. Jensen, S.H. Sandø, P.J. Jørgensen and S. Antonsen, Am. J. Publ. Health, 1989, 79, 1385.
7. D.B. Calne, A. Eisen, E. McGreer and P. Spencer, Lancet, 1986, 1, 1067.

8. J.P. Bosch, A. Saccaggi, A. Lauer, C. Ronco, M. Belledonne and S. Glabman, Am. J. Med., 1983, 75, 943.
9. C. Fletcher and R. Peto, Br. Med. J., 1977, 2, 1645.
10. M.F.W. Festing, CRC Crit.Rev.Toxicol., 1987, 18, 1.

Heavy Metals in the General Population: Trend Evaluation and Interrelation with Trace Elements

B. Heinzow, H. Jessen, S. Mohr, and D. Riemer

INSTITUTE OF ENVIRONMENTAL TOXICOLOGY, FLECKENSTR. 4, D-2300 KIEL, GERMANY

1 INTRODUCTION

Anthropogenic pollution of the environment by organic and inorganic substances has been steadily increasing in the past. Several associated problems have been identified and countermeasures have been taken such as reduction of lead in petrol or emission limits for waste incineration and industrial discharge. Global environmental and biological monitoring of important pollutants and investigation of possible deleterious effects is required to curb the problems of pollution. Biomonitoring of heavy metals in the general population has the aim to assess exposure and regional and temporal influences thereupon. The Institute of Environmental Toxicology has conducted several studies during the past ten years in Slesvig-Holstein, the northern federal state of Germany. The results of the latest studies are presented in the following.

2 MATERIAL AND METHODS

Persons selected at random from the general population (poll-register) were asked for voluntary cooperation. Blood and urine samples were collected, citrated or acidified and stored frozen or at 4°C until analysis. A questionnaire and interview for assessment of demographic variables, life style, health status and occupation was part of the study.

Analytical procedure. Heavy metals and trace elements were analyzed by means of atomic absorption spectrometry with a Perkin-Elmer AAS 4000 and since 1989 with a PE-Zeeman AAS 5100 either with a graphite furnace or hydride system MHS 20.

Standard sample preparation and analytical methods were applied, analytical quality was assured by use of reference materials: Lanonorm control blood (Behring) and

Seronorm (Nycomed). Quality assurance also involved participation in the yearly QC-exercises of the German Association of Occupational Medicine (Hamburg, Erlangen, FRG).

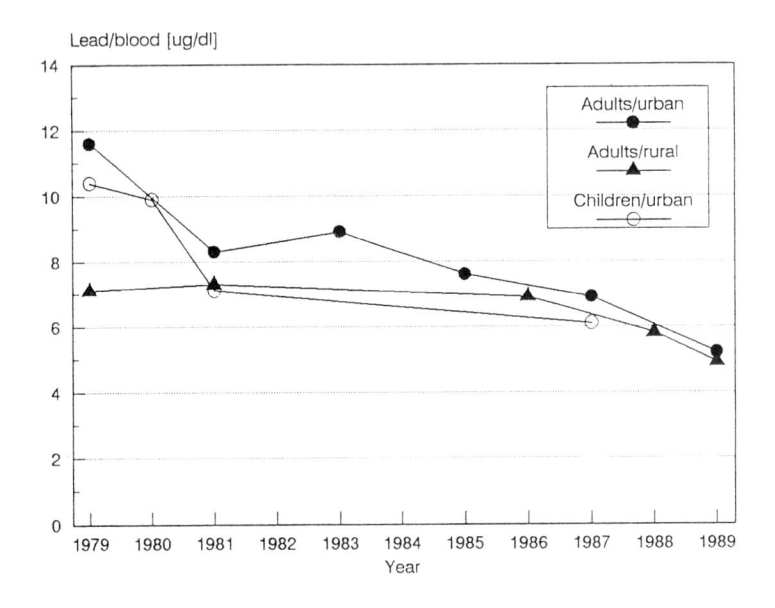

Fig 1. Time trend for lead in blood in adults and children (Slesvig-Holstein 1979-1989)

3 RESULTS AND DISCUSSION

Lead

Blood lead is a good indicator of current exposure and preferably used for studies of the general population[1]. Due to regulatory measures the pollution from leaded petrol and industrial emisson is declining. Since most of the foodstuff contamination is due to external deposition rather than soil-plant transfer the human external exposure is declining. The time trend of lead in blood of adults and children in Slesvig-Hostein shows a steady decline (Fig. 1). At present there is no significant difference between urban and rural areas. Blood lead levels above 15 µg/100mL in adults (Fig. 2) and 10 µg/100mL in children are seldom exceeded and should be further investigated to identify the individual source. With declining levels in the environment there is a greater chance to identify hidden sources in the vicinity such as soil contamination, drinking-water lead pipes and lead paint. The CEC reference values[2] from 1986 are at present no longer suitable for Northern Europe and should be adjusted to the current situation. Recent findings of neuropsychological effects of low level lead exposure[3] warrant a cautious approach to the acceptable lead burden in children.

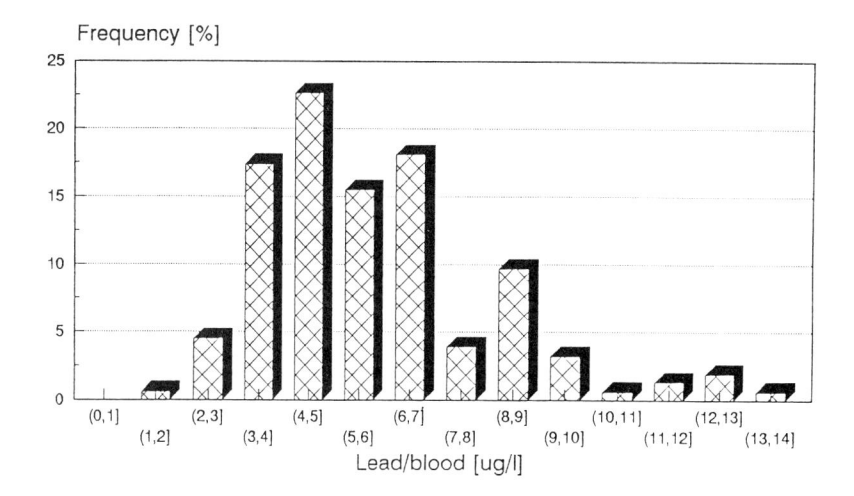

Fig. 2. Frequency distribution of lead in blood in adults
(Lägerdorf 1988)

Cadmium

In areas without heavy industrial pollution the cadmium exposure is mainly influenced by the personal smoking habits[4]. Smoking results in significantly higher blood cadmium levels, whereas in non-smokers 1,5 µg Cd/L blood are seldom exceeded (Fig. 3).

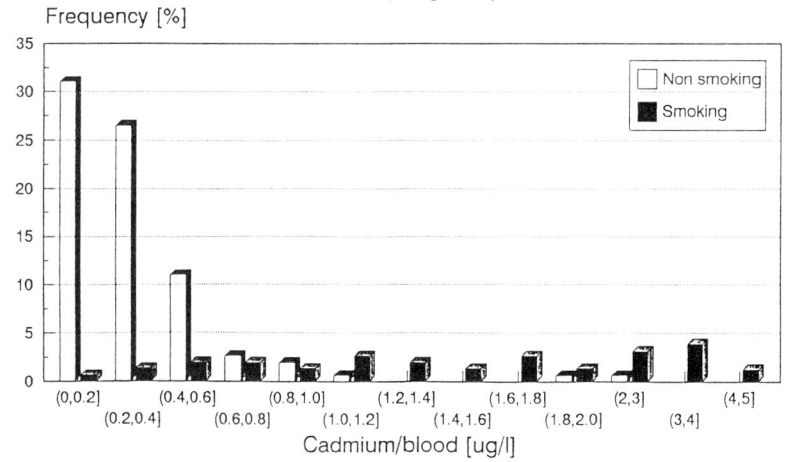

Fig. 3. Influence of smoking on blood cadmium levels in adults
(Lägerdorf 1988)

Mercury

Mercury in blood is clearly influenced by fish consumption (Table 1), with significantly elevated mean values in persons eating seafood once a week or more often. The ratio between mercury in blood (B-Hg) and serum (S-Hg) (Table 2) indicates that organic mercury is the dominant compound. Regional differences cannot be attributed solely to nutrional sources. There seems to be an increase in B-Hg in both the fish eating and non-fish eating population related to the area of residence close to the North Sea. Adults living in Flensburg, located at the Baltic Sea and Lägerdorf in the inland of Slesvig-Holstein have lower B-Hg exposure compared to St. Margret and Brunsbüttel at the west coast and Amrum, a North Sea island. A similar geographic gradient towards the Atlantic has been observed[5], however no data on fish consumption were given by the authors.

Table 1: Influence of fish-consumption on blood mercury in the general population from different regions in Slesvig-Holstein (Mean SD, µg/L)

Area	Rural/ urban	Fish consumption seldom	(n)	weekly	(n)
St. Margret	r	3.6 ± 4.7	(89)	5.7 ± 7.2	(62)
Brunsbüttel	u	2.1 ± 2.1	(37)	4.5 ± 3.8	(45)
Lägerdorf	r	2.2 ± 5.1	(81)	2.9 ± 2.8	(69)
Flensburg	u	0.4 ± 0.4	(43)	1.0 ± 0.9	(43)

Amalgam tooth fillings are of continous concern, Hahn and coworkers[6] have shown that dental amalgam can be a major source of chronic mercury exposure. In our latest study in 1989 there was no correlation between Hg in blood or serum but a weak association between the number of

Table 2 Biomotoring of heavy metals in the general population, Brunsbüttel 1989 (µg/L, n = 241 adults)

Element/Medium	Mean	Median	95 Perc.	Max.
Lead/Blood	51.0	45.0	97.0	203.0
Cadmium/Blood	0.5	0.3	1.6	4.4
Cadmium/Urine	0.3	0.2	0.8	1.3
Mercury/Blood	4.1	2.2	14.0	39.8
Mercury/Serum	0.9	0.7	2.8	7.8
Mercury/Urine	0.8	0.5	2.6	8.0

amalgam fillings and U-Hg (Spearman, rank corr. r = 0,36, p < 0.001). It is concluded that a single determination of Hg in blood or serum is not suitable for solving amalgam related complaints. Recent results with mobilisation of mercury stored in kidney by DMPS (Dimaval)[7] should be pursued to resolve the open questions about health and dental amalgam.

Selenium

Correlations of the concentrations of essential trace elements copper, zinc and selenium in blood were studied with the internal exposure of the heavy metals. No correlation was observed for zinc and copper in serum and the other compounds. Selenium is correlated to blood and serum mercury. Great geographic variation of the soil content do exist for Se and consequently through the food chain in human blood levels from different regions. Despite low or deficient soil concentrations in Northern Germany[8], the blood levels of the general population range from 60 to 140 µg Se/L blood (Fig. 4), which is regarded as safe. This is most likely related to the homogeneous nutrition with widely distributed and imported foodstuff and feed and rare exclusive supply of meat, grain and dairy products from local farmers. Hence availability of Se is greater than anticipated from local soil content.

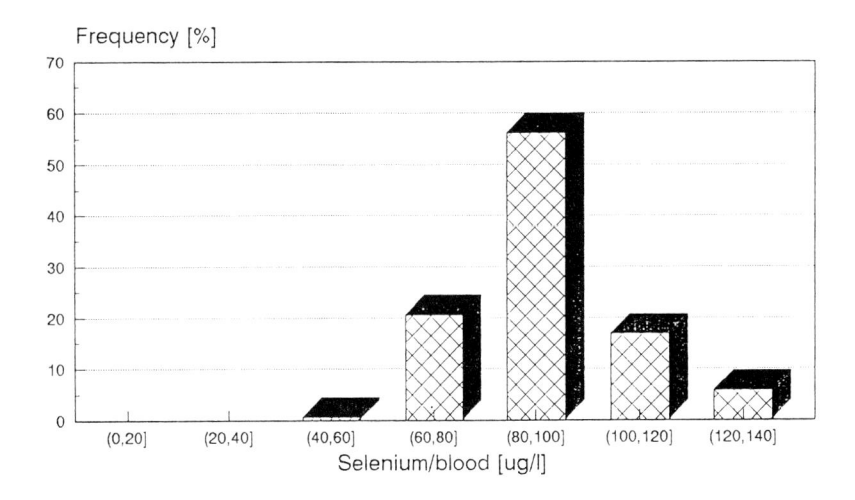

Fig 4. Frequency distribution of selenium in blood in adults (Lägerdorf 1988)

An interesting observation was made in all studies upon the interrelation between Se and Hg in blood (Fig. 5). There seems to be a general but region-specific correlation between these elements, which is not related to a common nutritional source. It is speculated that Hg-exposure is related to fish consumption and geographic region and that selenium affects the distribution of mercury in the organism.

Mercury/blood [ug/l] (Mean, S.D.)

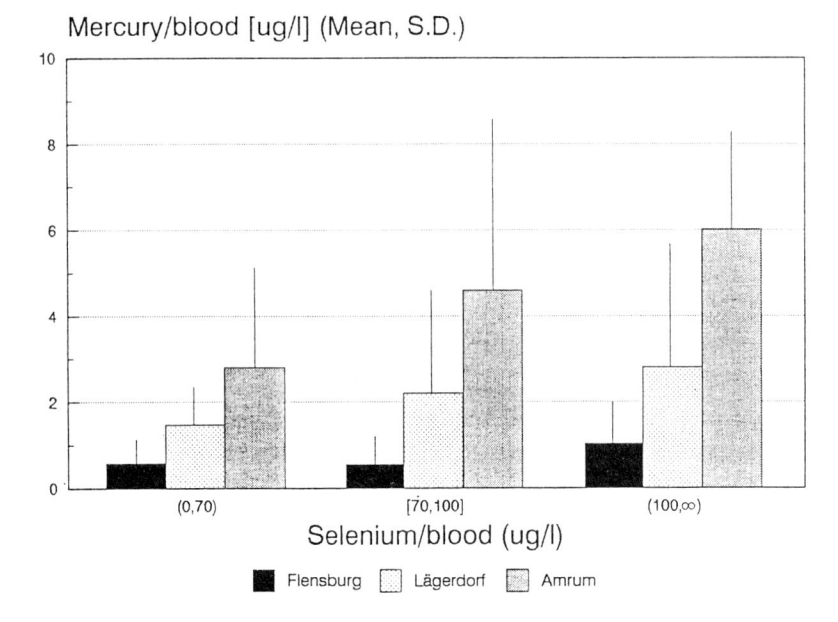

[Bar chart with x-axis labeled Selenium/blood (ug/l) with categories (0,70), [70,100], (100,∞); legend: Flensburg, Lägerdorf, Amrum]

Fig 5. Concentration of mercury in blood in people with different blood selenium concentrations in three districts in Germany.

4 CONCLUSION

In summary our results indicate temporal (Pb), regional (Hg) and individual (Cd) factors influencing the exposure of the general population with heavy metals. It is concluded that a region specific approach (cadaster) and temporal update of reference values is superior for evaluation, sources identification and reduction in environmental medicine.

For Northern Germany we propose the following regional reference values for heavy metal concentrations in the blood, derived from the 95 percentile:

Element	Reference value (μg/L)	Comment
Lead	100	Children
Lead	150	Adults
Cadmium	1.5	Nonsmokers
Mercury	5	Seldom fish

5 ACKNOWLEDGEMENT

We wish to thank Mrs. Kirsten Hänel for preparing the graphics and the manuscript.

6 REFERENCES

1. M. Vahter, GEMS, Karolinska Institute, Stockholm, 1982.
2. A. Berlin and M. Th. v. d. Venne, Commission of the EC, Luxemburg CEC/LUX/V/E/3/14/86, 1986.
3. G. Raab et al., II. Nordic Trace Element Symposium, Odense 1987.
4. C. Grasmick and G. F. Huel, Sci. Tot. Environm., 1985, 41, 207.
5. C. Grasmick and G. F. Huel, Sci. Tot. Environm., 1985, 45, 101.
6. L. J. Hahn et al., FASEB J., 1989, 3, 2641.
7. R. Schiele, K. H. Schaller, D. Weltle, Arbeitsmed. Sozialmed. Präventivmed., 1989, 24, 249.
8. W. Hartfiel and U. Bahners, VitaMinSpur, 1987, 2, 125.

Trace Element Levels in the Hair, Blood, Cord Blood and Placenta of Pregnant Women from Central Slovenia

M. Horvat, A. Prosenc, J. Smrke, D. Konda, A. R. Byrne, P. Stegnar, and I. Bergic[1]

J. STEFAN INSTITUTE, E. KARDELJ UNIVERSITY, LJUBLJANA, YUGOSLAVIA

[1] FACULTY OF MEDICINE, E. KARDELJ UNIVERSITY, LJUBLJANA, YUGOSLAVIA

1 INTRODUCTION

In recent years there has been considerable interest in studying the toxic effects and role of some essential trace elements during pregnancy. Among the toxic elements, mercury and especially methyl-Hg has been the most extensively investigated since it passes the placental barrier and is accumulated in the foetus. On the basis of mercury levels in human hair found so far, the Yugoslav population from the coastal regions has not been considered to be at risk[1,2]. This was further confirmed on the basis of a study of pregnant women and foetuses from the Central Adriatic Islands, who were known to be exposed to methyl-Hg due to higher seafood consumption[3]. In order to find a control group for the above mentioned study, pregnant women from Central Slovenia remote from the sea, who were absolutely non-seafood eaters were selected for the present study, and relationships between concentrations of total and methyl mercury in various samples were investigated.

2 MATERIALS AND METHODS

All studied samples together with information considered useful for the interpretation of data (age, location, occupation, number of amalgam fillings, smoking, nutritional habits) were taken at the time of birth in the Maternity Hospital in Ljubljana. Only pregnant women who were absolutely non-seafood eaters were included.

Hair samples were cleaned and stored according to IAEA recommendations[4]. Only the first cm of occipital hair was taken for analysis. Maternal blood was collected by venipuncture. Umbilical cord and maternal blood were heparinized, plasma and erythrocytes were separated immediately after sampling and stored at -20°C in precleaned polyethylene tubes until analysed. Amnion and chorion were separated and two placental compartments containing blood, the central part and the peripheral part, were taken. Samples were placed in precleaned

Table 1. Concentration of total and methylmercury in hair (µg/g) and blood components (ng/mL) from pregnant women from Central Slovenia (Control), seafood consuming women (from ref. 3), and women from mercury mining area.

Tissue	Control group, n=17 Total Hg Mean SD (range)	Control group, n=17 Methyl Hg Mean SD (range)	Control group, n=17 % MeHg Mean SD (range)	Seafood consumers (ref.3), n=34 Total Hg Mean SD (range)	Seafood consumers (ref.3), n=34 Methyl Hg Mean SD (range)	Seafood consumers (ref.3), n=34 % MeHg Mean SD (range)	Hg-mining area, (n=3) Total Hg	Hg-mining area, (n=3) MeHg	Hg-mining area, (n=3) MeHg %
Scalp hair	0.17 0.09 (0.08–0.35)	0.15 0.07 (0.08–0.34)	88 13 (63–100)	1.48 0.71 (0.42–3.28)	1.15 0.66 (0.20–3.36)	72 17 (40–100)	0.16 0.24 0.88	0.15 0.20 0.84	94 83 95
Pubic hair	0.15 0.06 (0.07–0.30)	0.14 0.07 (0.07–0.36)	85 14 (57–100)	1.39 0.80 (0.55–3.04)	1.11 0.69 (0.41–2.90)	79 18 (33–100)	0.25 0.22 0.85	0.18 0.22 0.84	71 100 99
Maternal blood	1.02 0.41 (0.24–1.63)	0.45 0.23 (0.14–0.90)	46 17 (19–72)	3.7 1.9 (1.2–9.6)	3.1 1.2 (0.3–7.9)	73 29 (21–100)	6.85 2.86 3.57	0.30 0.52 1.57	4.5 18 44
Maternal plasma	0.82 0.57 (0.06–2.44)	0.13 0.08 (0.01–0.31)	20 14 (1.3–49)				8.90 3.65 1.63	0.13 0.16 0.82	1.5 4.5 50
Maternal erythrocytes	1.29 0.75 (0.32–2.45)	0.74 0.37 (0.07–1.35)	71 43 (7–100)				9.59 2.81 6.41	0.42 1.24 5.45	4.3 44 85
Cord blood	1.16 0.80 (0.29–3.80)	0.74 0.35 (0.29–1.61)	77 36 (26–100)	7.7 5.1 (1.2–21.1)	6.7 4.8 (0.8–21.3)	80 19 (43–100)	4.30 2.25 6.11	0.64 1.31 4.60	15 58 75
Cord plasma	0.55 0.28 (0.06–1.20)	0.19 0.10 (0.01–0.41)	34 21 (1–86)				2.16 1.20 1.04	0.30 0.26 1.02	14 21 98
Cord erythrocytes	1.28 1.25 (0.60–5.92)	1.21 0.39 (0.45–2.00)	76 33 (33–100)				5.23 2.81 8.89	1.11 2.64 7.39	21 94 83

Table 2. Concentration of total and methylmercury in placenta, amnion and chorion (ng/g dry weight) from pregnant women from Central Slovenia (Control), seafood consuming women (from ref. 3), and women from mercury mining area.

Tissue	Control group, n=17 Total Hg Mean SD (range)	Control group, n=17 Methyl Hg Mean SD (range)	Control group, n=17 %MeHg Mean SD (range)	Seafood consumers, n=34 Total Hg Mean SD (range)	Seafood consumers, n=34 Methyl Hg Mean SD (range)	Seafood consumers, n=34 %MeHg Mean SD (range)	Hg-mining area, (n = 3) Total Hg	Hg-mining area, (n = 3) MeHg	Hg-mining area, (n = 3) MeHg %
Central placenta	14.5 5.0 (5.1-24.1)	2.9 1.3 (0.55-5.6)	21 12 (5-57)	72 43 (16-207)	39 28 (8-142)	56 26 (10-100)	112 40 59	2.74 2.40 17.6	2 6 30
Peripheral placenta	13.7 7.4 (1.5-35.1)	2.9 1.4 (0.57-6.07)	27 21 (4-82)	74 39 (24-171)	37 261 (9-122)	50 23 (14-100)	147 73 55	2.2 1.40 12.1	2 2 22
Amnion	21.3 12.6 (6.2-57.1)	6.80 3.30 (2.7-13.2)	35 17 (10-62)				74 64 51	2.80 5.90 51	4 10 100
Chorion	30.4 13.0 (13.5-63.1)	7.40 4.70 (2.5-20.4)	25 12 (6-48)				165 114 45	3.73 5.21 44.8	2 5 99

polyethylene containers and stored in freezer until analysed.

Total mercury in hair was determined by cold vapour atomic absorption (CVAAS)[5], and in all other samples total mercury and selenium were determined simultaneously by radiochemical neutron activation analysis (RNAA)[6,7]. Methyl-Hg in hair samples was determined by volatilization, isolation and gas chromatography with electron-capture detection (GC-ECD)[8,9], and in all other samples by ion-exchange and CVAAS[10]. Cu, Zn, As and Sb were determined by RNAA[11,12].

3 RESULTS AND DISCUSSION

The accuracy and precision of the analytical results obtained for Hg, Cu, Zn, As and Sb were checked by the analysis of certified or standard reference materials (CRMs/SRMs). The accuracy of the analytical methodology for methyl-Hg was assured by analysis of CRMs (National Research Council of Canada), interlaboratory comparisons, standard addition experiments and comparison of the results obtained by different techniques, which have been described elsewhere[13,14]. As methylmercury concentrations in blood, placenta and foetal membranes were very low, and sample weights small, we chose the ion-exchange separation technique in combination with gold amalgamation CVAAS with a detection limit of 0.01 ng Hg/g.

Mean values and ranges of concentrations of total and methyl-Hg in all samples examined are presented in Tables 1 and 2. For comparison, results from our previous study on seafood eaters are also presented. It is evident that concentrations of total and methyl-Hg in all samples are much lower in the control group than in the seafood-eating group, which indicates that a good control group was selected. Among 20 women, three were from a mercury mining area and consequently they showed much higher mercury levels in blood and especially in placental and foetal membrane compartments. Therefore the results for mercury and methyl-Hg in these women are presented separately from the control group, but according to the variability of the percentage of methyl-Hg in their blood and placental compartments, further studies should be done on this group.

No correlations between the number of amalgam fillings (the number varied between 1 to 16) and total mercury concentrations in the samples analysed were observed in the control group.

In general, good correlations between various samples from an individual were observed for methyl-Hg, but not for total mercury. The positive correlation ($r=0.62$, $p<0.05$) between methyl-Hg in scalp hair and maternal blood again proves the suitability of scalp hair in assessing methyl-Hg exposure. A good correlation between methyl-Hg in scalp and pubic hair was found (r=0.80, p<0.01), which again leads us to the conclusion that pubic hair could also be used as an indicator tissue. The cord blood/maternal blood methyl-Hg relationship is presented in Fig. 1, indicating higher concentrations in cord blood even at such low concentration levels. Total mercury in cord plasma is lower than in maternal plasma, which is in agreement with some other studies[15], while methyl-Hg in maternal and cord plasma are in good correlation (r=0.79, p<0.01); and are not significantly different from each other.

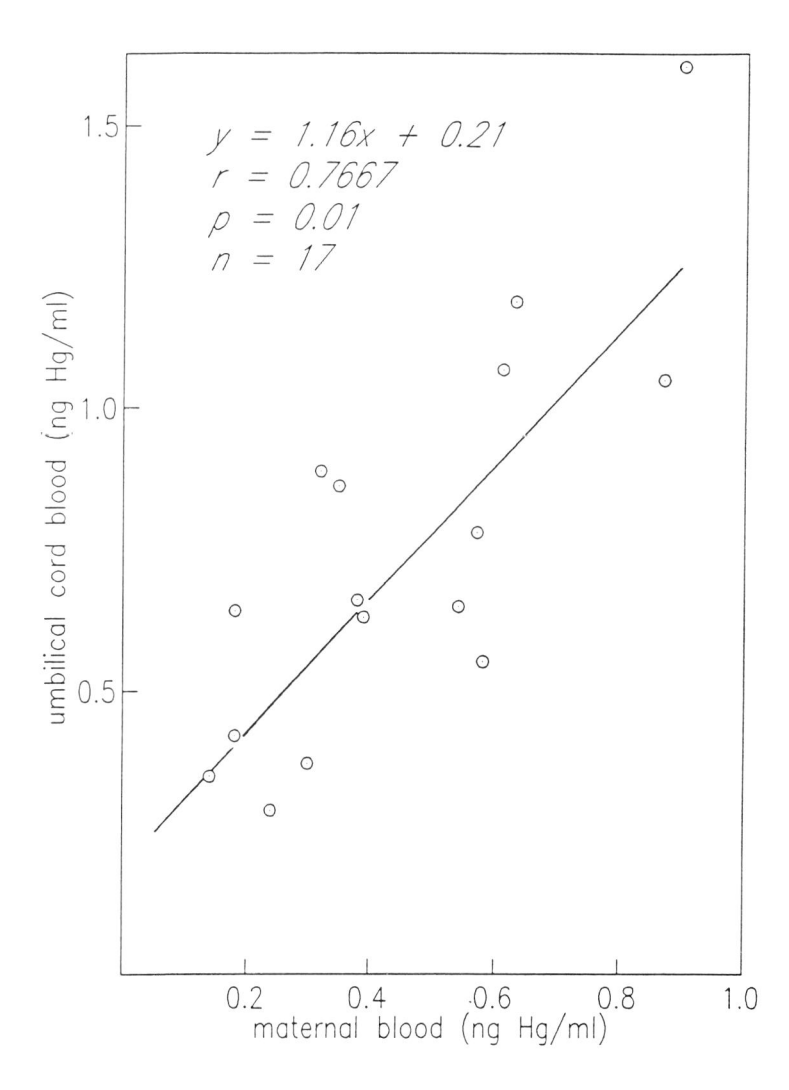

Fig 1. Correlation between methylmercury concentrations in **maternal** and cord blood.

Total and methyl-Hg levels are higher in foetal membranes than in the blood-containing parts of the placenta. Total mercury is significantly higher in chorion than in amnion, but no difference was found for methyl-Hg. No significant correlations between total Hg levels in various compartments of the placenta with the other samples analysed were found. In contrast, strong correlations between methyl-Hg in amnionic and chorionic membranes (r=0.89, p<0.001), and central and peripheral blood containing placenta (r=0.83, p<0.001) were found. The percentages of methyl-Hg in placental compartments are lower in the control group than in the seafood consuming group, and therefore it would be of interest to investigate whether placental and foetal membranes can be used as an indicator in assessing the type of mercury exposure during pregnancy.

Table 3 Concentrations of arsenic in maternal and cord blood components (ng/mL), and the placenta (ng/g dry weight), of Central Slovenian (Control) women, and of seafood consumers (from reference [3])

Tissue	Control population				Seafood consumers (Ref. 3)			
	N	Mean	SD	Range	N	Mean	SD	Range
Maternal								
blood	6	1.08	0.94	0.22-2.70	26	11.6	8.8	0.9-28.9
plasma		1.13	1.05	0.13-2.79				
erythrocytes		0.71	0.36	0.34-1.22				
Cord								
blood	6	1.18	0.89	0.18-2.52	26	8.0	7.5	0.9-31.0
plasma		1.21	0.53	0.68-2.03				
erythrocytes		0.87	1.02	0.21-2.94				
Placenta								
Central	16	2.62	1.66	1.03-8.00	34	32.5	29.0	4.0-113
Peripheral	15	2.96	1.11	1.34-4.70		28.5	26.5	5.0-100
Amnion	16	21.8	34.5	1.66-109				
Chorion	17	6.28	4.38	0.91-14.8				

The fact that methyl-Hg concentrations are higher in cord blood, and the percentage of methyl-Hg in cord blood compartments is higher than in maternal blood, together with the low percentage of methyl-Hg in placenta and foetal membranes and the good correlations between methyl-Hg levels within the placental compartments confirm the placental transfer of methyl-Hg and suggest removal of inorganic Hg before it can be transferred to the foetus.

Comparison of the results for arsenic in the control group and the seafood consuming group are presented in Table 3. It is evident that As is much lower in the control group in all samples analysed, which is the consequence of the high arsenic content of the seafood diet. A strong correlation (r=0.94, p<0.001) between As levels in maternal and cord blood was found. Arsenic levels in amnionic membrane are higher than in any other placental compartment. We were unable to compare these results to other studies since to the best of our knowledge, there are no data in the literature on the ability of As to cross the human placenta.

Table 4. Concentrations of selenium, copper, zinc and antimony in maternal blood, cord blood and placenta of Central Slovenian women

Tissue	Selenium µg/L Mean SD (Range)	Copper mg/L Mean SD (Range)	Zinc mg/L Mean SD (Range)	Antimony µg/L Mean SD (Range)
Maternal blood	98 61 (39-229) [n=18]	1.36 0.19 (1.07-1.55) [n=5]	4.31 1.30 (3.23-6.52) [n=5]	
plasma	63 34 (14-139) [n=18]	1.60 0.42 (1.17-2.17) [n=5]	0.57 0.08 (0.45-0.67) [n=5]	
erythrocytes	101 36 (48-157) [n=19]	0.63 0.22 (0.43-1.09) [n=5]	7.81 1.49 (6.09-8.86) [n=5]	
Cord blood	76 35 (37-174) [n=18]	0.56 0.08 (0.38-0.60) [n=6]	2.02 0.57 (1.61-2.55) [n=5]	
plasma	87 76 (15-251) [n=18]	0.23 0.03 (0.20-0.27) [n=5]	0.62 0.06 (0.56-0.68) [n=5]	
erythrocytes	113 44 (28-213) [n=20]	0.64 0.05 (0.58-0.72) [n=6]	2.31 0.18 (0.99-2.62) [n=5]	
Placenta	ng/g	µg/g	µg/g	ng/g
central	839 246 (581-1282) [n=20]	4.03 0.81 (2.09-5.48) [n=19]	42.5 13.0 (14.1-65.3) [n=16]	1.44 0.90 (0.57-2.88) [n=6]
peripheral	892 133 (430-1222) [n=20]	4.96 1.70 (2.49-9.80) [n=18]	37.9 13.9 (17.7-63.4) [n=17]	5.22 7.21 (0.41-22.5) [n=8]
Amnion	571 291 (138-1195) [n=20]	5.85 5.36 (0.52-22.3) [n=18]	32.9 14.4 (13.6-68.5) [n=16]	10.1 7.9 (2.62-24.1) [n=8]
Chorion	1044 458 (497-1933) [n=20]	7.11 4.24 (1.94-17.5) [n=19]	32.6 20.9 (10.8-48.1) [n=17]	8.05 14.3 (1.20-48.3) [n=10]

Results for copper, zinc, selenium and antimony are presented in Table 4. Concentrations of Cu in blood and placenta samples lay within the range of normal pregnancy. Maternal plasma levels of copper were higher than normal plasma copper in nonpregnant women and cord plasma levels of copper were much lower than those of maternal plasma, which is in accordance with some other studies[16,17].

From the results for zinc in Table 4, it is evident that cord blood Zn levels lay within the range of normal pregnancy, but Zn levels in maternal blood compartments and placenta were slightly lower than reported in the literature[18]. This could be explained by the small number of samples analysed in this study.

Se levels are more variable than those of other essential trace elements since its concentration in blood is highly responsive to changes in the level in the diet. Erythrocytes contain higher selenium levels than plasma in maternal and cord blood. Good correlations ($r=0.94$, $p<0.001$) between Se levels in whole maternal blood and maternal plasma, and between Se levels in whole maternal blood and central placenta were found. No correlations were observed between Se levels in maternal and cord blood, or between mercury and selenium in any of the samples analysed.

The concentrations of antimony in blood samples were below the detection limit of the analytical method (0.01 ng/g), and therefore a few results for Sb in placental compartments only are presented in Table 4. Foetal membranes contain more Sb than the placenta containing blood, but the results could not be compared to any other study due to limited information about Sb in the normal human population.

To conclude, in this work, by examining a totally non-fish eating population, we have attempted to determine base-line levels of total and methyl mercury in hair, maternal and cord blood, and placental tissue for subjects with a minimal mercury intake. Such values should represent a useful basis for comparison with other populations and other types of exposure.

4 ACKNOWLEDGEMENTS

We gratefully acknowledge financial support of this study by the Research Community of Slovenia through the project "Microelements in Biological Tissues and Fluids". We thank Dr. A.Sabadin for statistical evaluation of the data.

5 REFERENCES

1. M.Dermelj, M.Horvat, A.R.Byrne and P.Stegnar, Chemosphere, 1986, 16, 887.
2. WHO/UNEP/FAO, Report on a joint WHO/UNEP/FAO Consultation Meeting on Mediterranean Health-Related Environmental Quality Criteria EUR/ICP/CEH 059(S), Bled, Yugoslavia, 1988.

3. M.Horvat, P.Stegnar, A.R.Byrne, M.Dermelj and Z.Branica, 'Trace Element Analytical Chemistry in Medicine and Biology', Walter de Gruyter & Co., Berlin.New York, 1988, 5, 243.
4. Ju.S. Rjabuchin, IAEA Report RL-50, Vienna, 1978.
6. M.Horvat, T.Zvonaric and P.Stegnar, Vestn. Slov. Kem.Drus., 1986, 33, 475.
7. L.Kosta and A.R.Byrne, Talanta, 1969, 16, 1297.
8 A.R.Byrne and L.Kosta, Talanta, 1973, 21, 1083.
9. V.Zelenko and L.Kosta, Talanta, 1973, 20, 115.
10. I.Gvardjancic, L.Zelenko and L.Kosta, Zh.Anal.Khim., 1978, 32, 812.
11. A.R.Byrne and A.Vakselj, Croat.Chem.Acta, 1974, 46, 225.
12. M.Dermelj, A.Vakselj, V.Ravnik and B.Smodis, Radiochem. Radioanal.Letters, 1979, 41, 149.
13. M.Horvat, K.May, M.Stoeppler and A.R.Byrne, Appl.Organomet. Chem., 1988, 2, 515.
14. M.Horvat, A.R.Byrne and K.May, Talanta, 1990, 37, 207.
15. A.Wannag and J.Skjaerasen, Environ. Physiol. Biochem., 1975, 5, 348.
16. W. Mertz, 'Trace elements in Human and Animal Nutrition', A.P.Inc., Fifth Edition, New York, 1986.
17. M. Abdulla, L.Löfberg, M. Jägerstad, I. Qvist, S. Svensson and A. Åberg, 'Trace Element Analytical Chemistry in Medicine and Biology', P. Brätter and P. Schramel, eds., Walter de Gruyter, Berlin and New York., 1983, 2, 517.
18. E. Damsgaard, K.Heydorn and N. Horn., 'Trace Element-Analytical Chemistry in Medicine and Biology', P. Brätter and P. Schramel, eds., Walter de Gruyter, Berlin, New York, 1983, 2, 499.

Kinetics of Heavy Metals

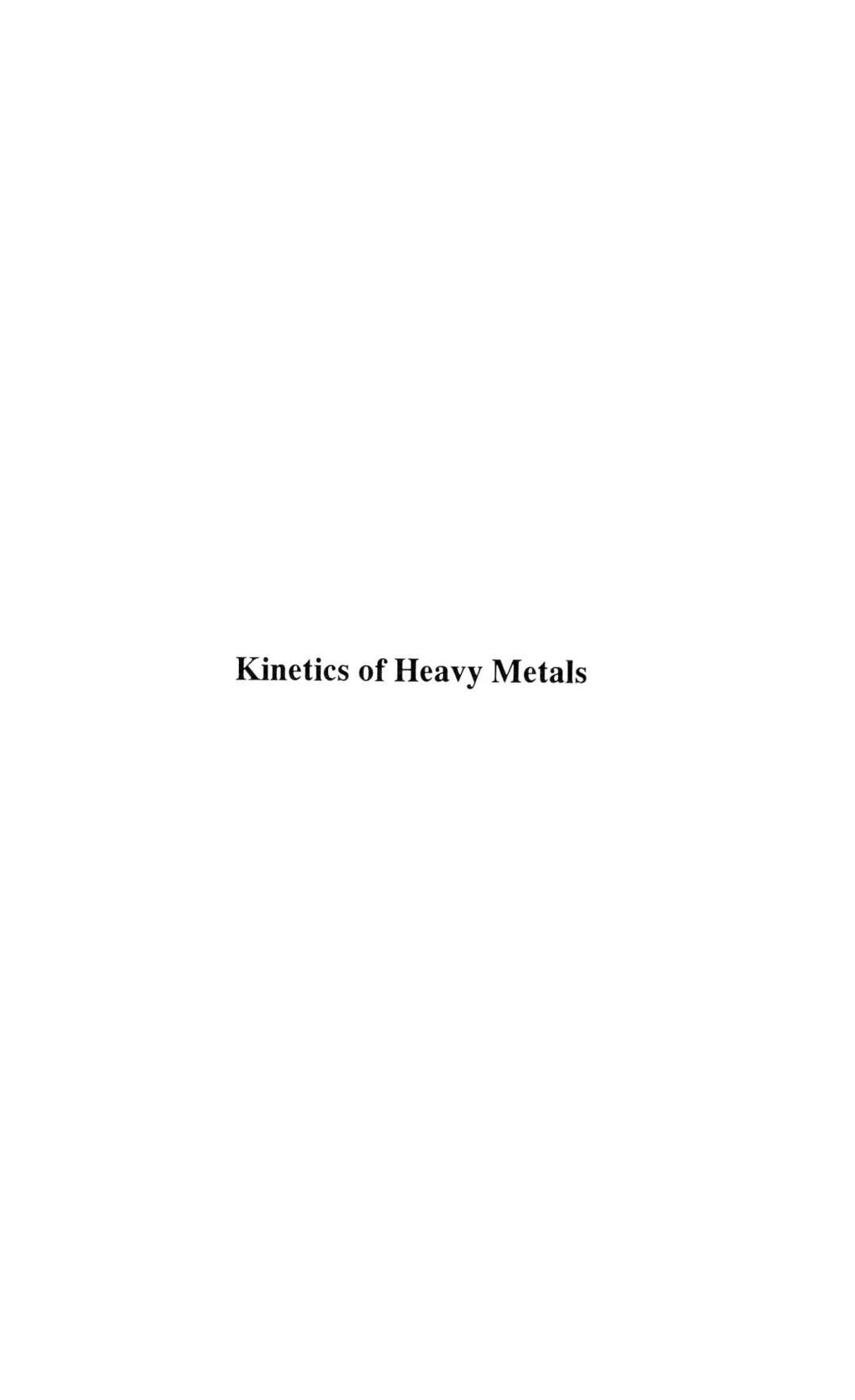

Cadmium Toxicokinetics Following Long-term Occupational Exposure

R. A. Braithwaite[1], R. Armstrong[2], D. M. Franklin[2,3], D. R. Chettle[2], and M. C. Scott[2]

[1] REGIONAL LABORATORY FOR TOXICOLOGY, DUDLEY ROAD HOSPITAL, BIRMINGHAM, B18 7QH, UK
[2] SCHOOL OF PHYSICS AND SPACE RESEARCH, UNIVERSITY OF BIRMINGHAM, B15 2TT, UK
[3] PRESENT ADDRESS: PATENTS DEPARTMENT, R.S.R.E.,MALVERN, WR14 3PS, UK

1 INTRODUCTION

Cadmium and its salts are widely used in many industries and the health risks associated with occupational exposure have been recognised for many years[1]. The major target organ associated with toxicity due to long-term exposure is the kidney[1]. Of particular interest is the renal tubular dysfunction, which is characterised by an increased excretion of low molecular weight proteins in urine such as β_2-microglobulin ($\beta_2 M$)[1]. However, the long-term effects of chronic cadmium exposure are difficult to assess due to the complexity of cadmium toxicokinetics[1-3]. In man, cadmium has an extremely long residence time (> 20 years) in the body, and a significant proportion of the body burden is stored in liver and kidney and bound to metallothionein[1]. Various kinetic models for cadmium have been described[3-4], but these are mostly based on limited human data or very short study periods. Long-term studies are required to investigate cadmium toxicokinetics in man and to make proper risk assessments.

The present study is unique, in that it combines *in vitro* measurements of cadmium in body fluids carried out over a prolonged period with *in vivo* measurements in tissues so as to gain a clearer insight of cadmium toxicokinetics following chronic exposure.

2 SUBJECTS

A group of 14 male workers (mean age 51, S.D. 14 years) who had been occupationally exposed in one factory to cadmium fume of varying intensity for periods of between 2 and 26 years (mean 15, S.D. 9 years) were the subjects of the investigation. All but one worker had been exposed to fume at or above the current U.K. occupational "limit" for cadmium in air (0.05 mg/m^3). All subjects gave their informed consent to the investigations which were carried out as part of the occupational health assessment that was supervised by the factory medical officer.

3 METHODS

Blood and urine specimens were obtained from each worker at approximately nine-monthly intervals between 1983 and 1989. In vivo measurement of liver and kidney cadmium was carried out at a single point late in 1983 in each subject using a neutron activation technique, which has previously been described[5-6]. All use of cadmium alloys was suspended in the factory following results of initial blood and urine tests that were also carried out during 1983. Blood and urinary cadmium concentrations were measured using electrothermal atomic absorption spectrometry, paying strict attention to accuracy control; urinary β_2M was measured in freshly voided specimens (without pH manipulation) using a radioimmunoassay procedure (Pharmacia, Sweden).

4 RESULTS

The distributions of values for the measurements of blood and urinary cadmium (Cd) at the start of the study are shown in Figures 1a and 1b respectively. The distributions of liver and kidney cadmium measured a few months later, at the end of 1983, are shown in Figures 2a and 2b respectively. The distribution of values for urinary β_2-microglobulin concentrations at the start of the study is shown in Figure 3.

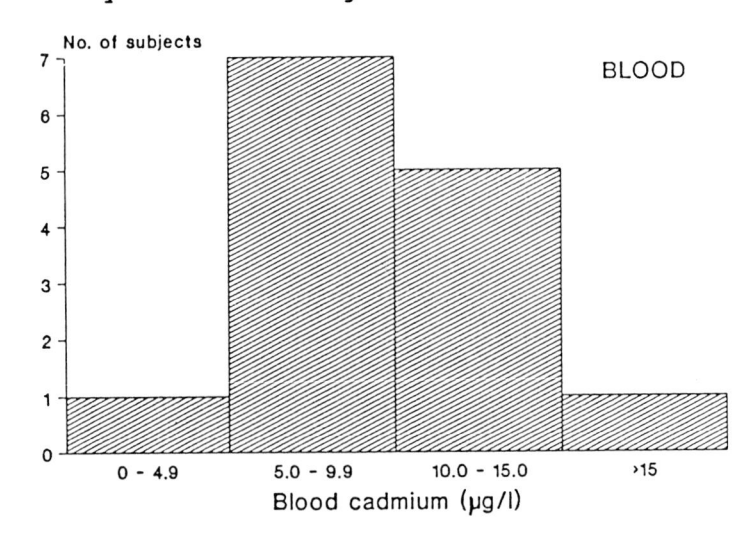

Figure 1a Distribution of cadmium in blood

From the distribution of values for urinary β_2M excretion it was possible to divide the subjects into two groups i.e. "normal" β_2M excretion in urine (<500 µg/g creatinine) and "elevated" β_2M excretion in urine (> 500 µg/g creatinine). Those subjects with an elevated excretion of β_2M in urine had statistically significantly higher mean concentrations of cadmium in blood, urine and liver, but not in kidney (Table 1). However, the range of kidney cadmium burdens in the "elevated" β_2M group (10-78 mg) was much larger than in the "normal" β_2M group (5-21 mg).

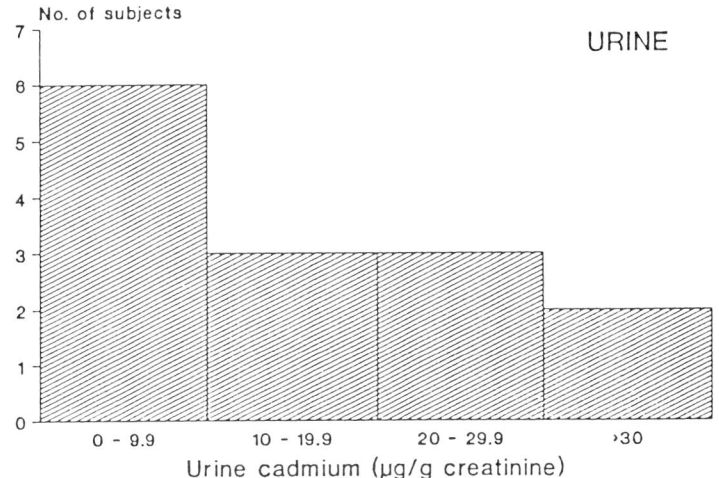

Figure 1b Distribution of cadmium in urine

The correlations between blood and urinary cadmium concentrations and liver and kidney cadmium burdens measured *in vivo* are shown in Table 2. In most cases there was a statistically significant correlation between *in vitro* and *in vivo* measurements. The strongest correlations were obtained between urinary cadmium concentration and kidney cadmium and estimated body burden of cadmium.

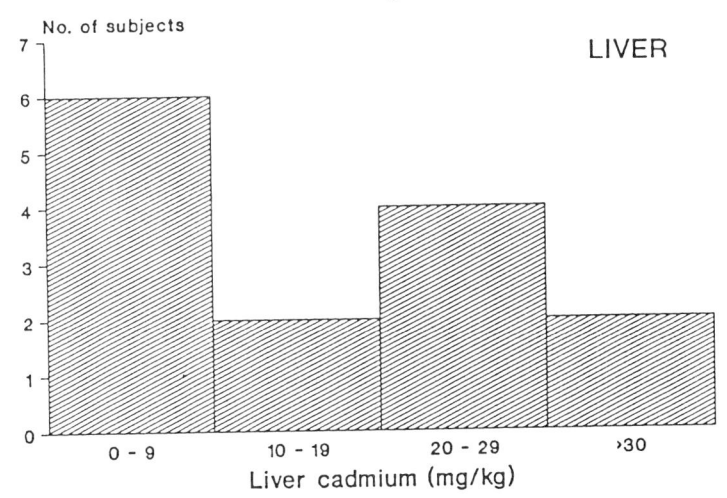

Figure 2a Distribution of cadmium in liver

KIDNEY

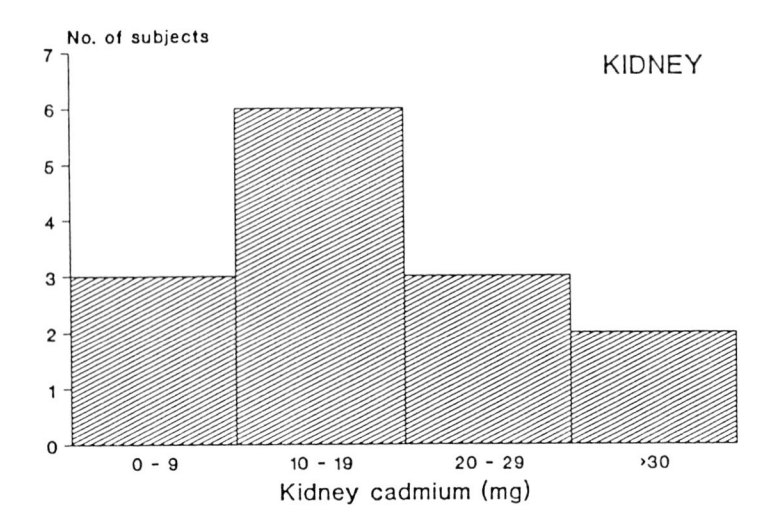

Figure 2b Distribution of cadmium in kidney

The changes in blood and urinary cadmium concentrations with time were plotted for each subject; an example of the decrease in urinary cadmium excretion with time for one subject is shown in Figure 4. The pattern of change for both blood and urinary cadmium appeared to differ between subjects with "normal" and those with raised β_2M excretion in urine. The urine cadmium excretion data for individual subjects were normalized by dividing each value by the calculated urinary cadmium concentration at the time of the *in vivo* measurement.

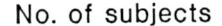

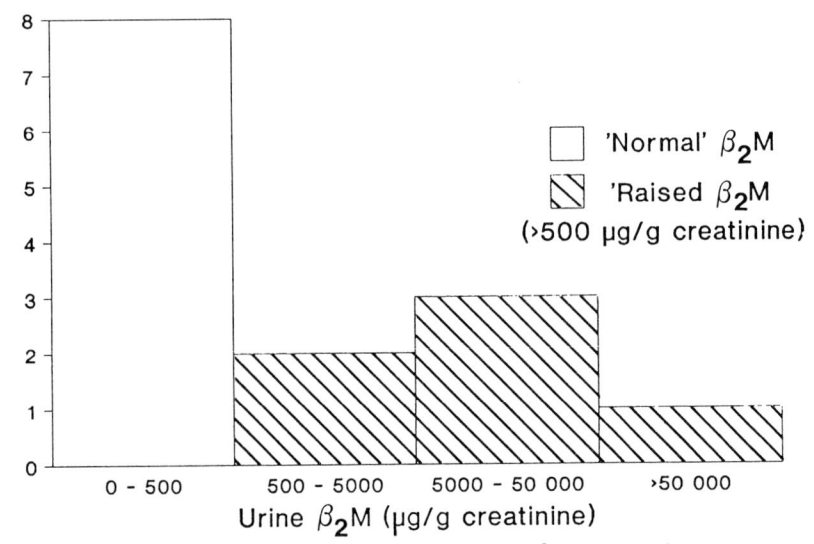

Figure 3 Distribution of urinary β_2M excretion

Table 1   Cadmium concentration in urine, blood, liver and kidney in subjects with normal and elevated $\beta_2 M$ excretion in urine (Mean (SD) is given)

Excretion of $\beta_2 M$	n	Blood Cd µg/L	Urinary Cd µg/g creatinine	Liver Cd mg/kg	Kidney Cd mg/kg
Normal (<500 µg/g creatinine)	8	6.4 (2.0)	6.7 (5.4)	9.3 (6.5)	12.3 (6.8)
Elevated (>500 µg/g creatinine)	6	12.2 (2.8)***	23.2 (8.5)***	33.2 (20.4)*	29.0 (25.1)
Total	14	9.5 (3.8)	16.4 (14.3)	19.5 (19.1)	19.4 (18.5)

* $p < 0.05$, *** $p < 0.001$

Table 2 Linear correlations (r) between blood and urinary cadmium (Cd) concentrations and measured in-vivo cadmium burdens in liver and kidney in subjects with "normal" and "elevated" $\beta_2 M$ excretion in urine

	Urinary Cd	Liver Cd	Kidney Cd	Body burden of Cd
Blood Cd				
Normal $\beta_2 M$	0.81*	0.57	0.90**	0.75*
Elevated $\beta_2 M$	0.68	0.91*	0.70	0.81
Urinary Cd				
Normal $\beta_2 M$	-	0.82*	0.95***	0.96***
Elevated $\beta_2 M$	-	0.92**	0.98***	0.97***
Kidney Cd				
Normal $\beta_2 M$	-	0.84**	-	-
Elevated $\beta_2 M$	-	0.91*	-	-

Body burden[4] = $\dfrac{1.8 \times \text{liver Cd} + 2 \times \text{kidney Cd}}{0.16 + 0.53}$ mg

Statistical significance:
* $p<0.05$, ** $p<0.01$, *** $p<0.001$

The normalized urinary cadmium data were considered in two groups for those subjects with "normal" and those with "elevated" $\beta_2 M$ excretion in urine. From these pooled data, an estimate of the mean elimination half-time for cadmium in urine was calculated for the two groups. In those subjects with an elevated β_2M excretion in urine, there was a statistically significant (r = 0.78, df = 34, p<0.001) mono-exponential loss of cadmium in urine with an estimated half-time of 5.2 (S.D. 0.6) years. For those subjects with a "normal" β_2M excretion in urine there was no statistically significant loss of cadmium in urine over the period of investigation. The changes in blood cadmium concentrations over the same period for both groups of subjects were less clear-cut.

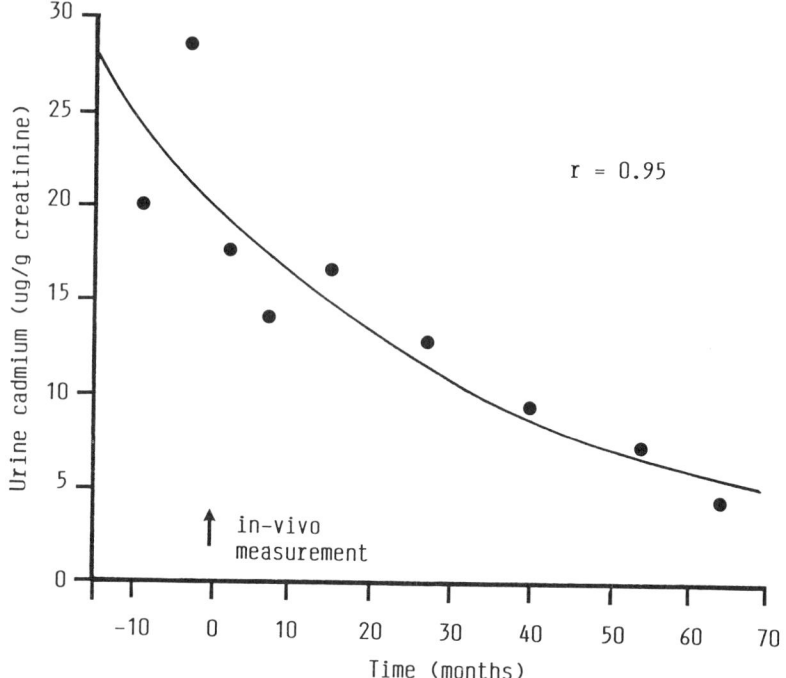

Fig 4. Urinary cadmium excretion after cessation of the exposure for one subject.

For each of the 5 subjects who had both an "elevated" excretion of β_2M in urine and a statistically significant loss of cadmium in urine with time, a one-compartment toxicokinetic model was considered. In this model, the size of the cadmium pool feeding the urinary cadmium excretion route was estimated from the fitted exponential excretion curve for each individual, assuming an average creatinine excretion of 1 g per day. The cadmium pool sizes were estimated for the time of the *in vivo* cadmium measurements and compared with the total kidney burden taken to be twice that of the measured *in vivo* cadmium content of the left kidney. Table 3 shows that the estimated and measured kidney cadmium burdens for these 5 subjects are in good agreement.

Table 3 Comparison between predicted and measured kidney cadmium burdens in five subjects, each with elevated urinary β_2M excretion, and a significant relationship between urinary cadmium excretion and time.

Subject no.	Kidney cadmium (mg) Predicted (S.D.)	Measured (S.D.)	Correlation coefficient*
9	54 (21)	30 (8)	0.87
11	68 (10)	62 (16)	0.96
12	12 (26)	20 (6)	0.85
13	29 (4)	32 (10)	0.95
14	72 (16)	48 (12)	0.88
TOTAL	235 (39)	192 (25)	

* $P < 0.05$ in each case.

5 DISCUSSION

Previously reported studies have indicated that liver cadmium is a much better index of cumulative cadmium exposure than is kidney cadmium[7,8]. The high values for liver cadmium found in the group with elevated urinary β_2M excretion indicates that they had accumulated significantly more cadmium than those subjects with normal β_2M excretion in urine (Table 1). Moreover, the mean duration of cadmium exposure in the elevated β_2M group was 16.1 years compared with only 4.8 years in the normal β_2M group. The finding that the kidney cadmium values for these two groups (Table 1) were not statistically different may be explained by the relative loss of kidney cadmium in those subjects with an elevated β_2M excretion and renal tubular damage; it is generally accepted that following the onset of damage, the kidney loses its ability to retain cadmium. These findings are also consistent with a statistically significantly greater urinary cadmium excretion in the group with an elevated β_2M excretion (Table 1).

A particularly strong correlation was obtained between urinary cadmium and kidney cadmium for both groups (Table 2). This suggests that when there is no current exposure, urinary cadmium reflects kidney cadmium both before and following the onset of renal tubular damage. This contrasts with the way in which urinary cadmium reflects current exposure following renal damage when exposure is continuing.[9] The gradient of the relationship between urine and kidney cadmium was significantly different (p<0.001) between the two groups, indicating a discontinuous relationship between kidney cadmium and urinary cadmium excretion.

From Table 2 it can be seen that blood cadmium shows a significant relationship with kidney cadmium in the normal β_2M group but not in the elevated β_2M group. Also, blood cadmium shows a significant relationship with liver cadmium in the elevated β_2M group, but not in the normal β_2M group. These findings are difficult to explain, but may indicate that the redistribution of cadmium between blood, liver and kidney stores may well be influenced by the onset of renal tubular damage and the length of time both during and after exposure. However, the size of the present study population may be too small to define this phenomenon more precisely.

This work has clearly shown that renal tubular function has a major influence on urinary cadmium excretion. In those subjects with normal β_2M excretion, there was only a small loss of cadmium in urine which showed no change over the duration of the study. In those subjects with elevated β_2M excretion, taken as indicative of renal tubular damage, the loss of cadmium in urine had an elimination half-time of approximately 5 years which is somewhat longer than previously described[4]. However, there have only been a limited number of earlier studies and these have been of shorter duration, which may explain their lower estimates of urinary cadmium elimination rate. Interestingly, there was a good agreement between measured and predicted values of kidney cadmium in those subjects with impaired tubular function (Table 3). This is perhaps surprising in view of the simplicity of the assumed model, and implies that the loss of cadmium via urine is mainly derived from kidney, rather than from blood or other stores. Further *in vivo* studies are planned in order to explore this finding.

The changes in blood cadmium concentration with time were on the whole less significant than those of urinary cadmium, and the distinction between the two groups was less marked. There was a trend towards a shorter blood elimination half-time in those subjects with normal β_2M excretion, but further studies are required to understand the pattern of change.

The present investigation has shown that the combined use of *in vitro* and *in vivo* techniques has proved to be a valuable tool for investigating cadmium toxicokinetics in man. It is hoped that the continuation of these studies will provide better insight into the problem.

6 ACKNOWLEDGEMENTS

We would like to thank Dr. S.S. Brown for valuable help and encouragement during this work. We would also like to thank Mrs. L.N. Mowen and Mrs. S. Clare for help in the preparation of this manuscript. We are also grateful to the Health and Safety Executive for financial support to RA, DMF and DRC.

7 REFERENCES

1. L. Friberg, T. Kjellstrom, G.F. Nordberg, "Handbook on the Toxicology of Metals - 2nd Edn. Vol. II Specific Metals", Elsevier Science Publishers, Amsterdam, 1986, p. 130.
2. H. Welinder, S. Skerfving and O. Henriksen, Brit. J. Ind. Med., 1977, 34, 221.
3. G.F. Nordberg and T. Kjellstrom, Environ. Health Persp. 1979, 28, 211.
4. G.F. Nordberg, T. Kjellstrom and M. Nordberg. Cadmium and Health: A Toxicological and Epidemiological Approach Vol. I. L. Friberg, C-G. Elinder, T. Kjellstrom, G.F. Nordberg (eds). CRC Press, Boca Raton, USA. 1985 p. 103.
5. J.G. Fletcher, D.R. Chettle and I.K. Al-Haddad, J. Radioanal. Chem. 1982, 71, 547.
6. M.C. Scott, and D.R. Chettle, Scand. J. Work Environ. Health, 1986, 2, 81.
7. H.J. Mason, A.G. Davison, A.L. Wright, C.J.G. Guthrie, P.M. Fayers, K.M. Venables, N.J. Smith, D.R. Chettle, D.M. Franklin, M.C. Scott, H. Holden, D. Gompertz and A.J. Newman-Taylor. Brit. J. Ind. Med. 1988, 45, 793.
8. K.J. Ellis, S.H. Cohn and T. Smith. J. Toxicol. Env. Health, 1985, 15, 173.
9. R.L. Lauwerys, J.P. Buchet, H. Roels, A. Bernard, D.R. Chettle, T.C. Harvey and I.K. Al-Haddad proc. 2nd Int. Cad. Conf. Metal Bulletin, London, 1980, p. 164.

Absorption of Bismuth from Two Bismuth Salts During *in Vivo* Perfusion of Rat Small Intestine

A. Slikkerveer, G. B. van der Voet, and F. A. De Wolff

TOXICOLOGY LABORATORY, UNIVERSITY HOSPITAL LEIDEN, PO BOX 9600, 2300 RC LEIDEN, THE NETHERLANDS

1 INTRODUCTION

The increasing use of colloidal bismuth subcitrate in the treatment of peptic ulcer and other *Helicobacter pylori*-related diseases has raised questions about the amount of bismuth (Bi) absorbed from the gastrointestinal tract and factors that influence this absorption. Knowledge of the amount of Bi absorbed could be an important guide to assess the exposure of patients to Bi after receiving Bi-containing drugs. After oral administration of Bi compounds a small but significant increase in blood Bi concentration has been observed.[1-3] Enhanced absorption has been demonstrated by 3-mercaptopropionic acid, cysteine and other sulphydryl group containing compounds.[4] The small intestine has been proposed as the site of absorption[5,6], but data on the exact localization of the absorption is still scanty. This experiment studied the concentration dependence of the absorption of Bi from bismuth chloride ($BiCl_3$) and colloidal bismuth subcitrate in the small intestine *in vivo*.

2 MATERIALS AND METHODS

Experiments were performed with female Wistar rats (200-220 g) fed on a standard diet (Hope farms, Woerden, The Netherlands) with tap water *ad libitum*. The rats had fasted 24 h before the experiment. An *in vivo* perfusion model[7] of the rat small intestine was used in combination with systemic blood sampling from the carotid artery. An isotonic medium containing Bi was recirculated through duodenum, ileum and jejunum at a perfusion rate of 10 mL/min. $BiCl_3$ was solubilized in citrate buffer (0.1 mol/L; pH 6.3) at concentrations of 0, 10, 100 and 1000 mg/L Bi^{3+}. Colloidal solutions of Bi subcitrate (CBS) in isotonic sodium chloride were also prepared in multiples of 10 from 10 to 100,000 mg/L CBS (bismuth subcitrate contains 35% Bi^{3+}). The exposure of the rat to soluble Bi was maximized by direct instillation of the solutions in the small intestine.

Samples of the perfusate (1 mL) and blood (100 µL) were collected for 60 min at 15 min intervals. Perfusate samples were diluted with 26 mmol/L HNO_3 and analysed by electrothermal atomic absorption spectrometry (EAAS). Blood samples were pipetted directly into 2% Triton X-100 with ammonium pyrrolidine dithiocarbamate and analysed after extraction. Intestinal absorption was measured as the appearance of Bi in blood at t = 60 min. The retention was defined as the decrease in the bismuth concentrations in the perfusate between t = 0 and t = 60 min. For all concentrations four or more experiments were performed.

3 RESULTS

The intestinal absorption was shown to be dependent on the concentration of $BiCl_3$ in the citrate buffer (Fig 1A) and CBS in isotonic sodium chloride (Fig 1B); a distinct increase in the blood concentration was observed when the perfusate concentration was raised. A blood concentration of 83 ± 5 µg/L Bi was found at t = 60 min for 1000 mg/L CBS and of 1416 ± 1250 µg/L (n=4) after perfusion with 1000 mg/L Bi^{3+} from $BiCl_3$. Absorption increased with perfusion time for both solutions. The retention of Bi by the intestinal mucosa from both solutions was also concentration dependent (Fig 1C and D). The magnitude of retention was in the millimolar range, while in blood Bi was present in micromolar amounts. The biological variation was large.

4 DISCUSSION

Intestinal absorption of Bi from Bi-containing medication may well be an important route of exposure for humans; the small intestine being a likely site of absorption. In this experiment Bi was indeed absorbed from the small intestine. It cannot be ruled out, however, that absorption of bismuth could also occur by the stomach mucosa. After oral intake of Bi compounds in man most of the Bi will precipitate in the stomach as insoluble salts (eg, BiOCl)[8], thus leaving an unknown, but possibly very small soluble fraction available for absorption. Even under the optimized conditions of this experiment the availability of the metal for absorption in the small intestine was very low.

Only a small concentration range could be used for $BiCl_3$ because of limited solubility of Bi in citrate buffer. The preparation of clear, isotonic perfusion solutions with a pH between four and seven for $BiCL_3$ was only possible in the presence of citrate; bismuth subcitrate formed a soluble colloid. It is suggested that the presence of citrate in both perfusion media played a role in the solubility of Bi compounds and may be involved in the mechanism of absorption itself.

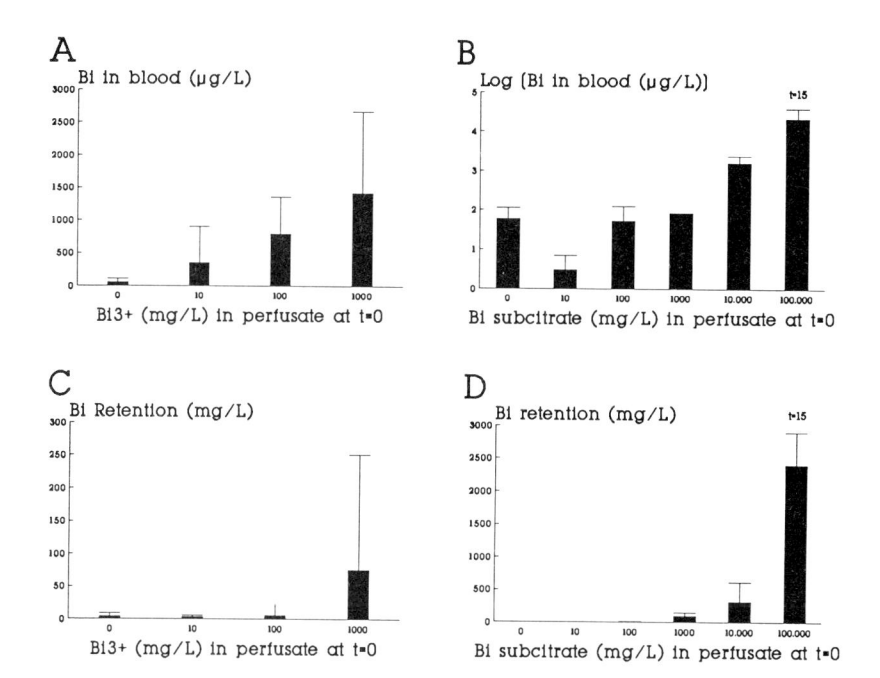

Fig 1. Absorption of bismuth at t = 60 min and retention of Bi after intestinal perfusion with two bismuth compounds. A: Absorption after perfusion with $BiCl_3$ in citrate buffer; B: Absorption after perfusion with CBS; C: Retention after perfusion with $BiCl_3$ in citrate buffer; D: Retention after perfusion with CBS. Note the logarithmic scale on the Y-axis in B.

5 REFERENCES

1. F. Conso, R. Bourdon and M. Gaultier, Eur. J. Toxicol., 1975, 8, 137.
2. D.W. Thomas, S. Sobecki, T.F. Hartley, P. Coyle and M.H. Alp, 'Chemical Toxicology and Clinical Chemistry of Metals', S.S. Brown and J. Savory, eds, Academic Press, London, 1983, p. 391.
3. S.P. Lee, Res. Commun. Chem. Pathol. Pharmacol., 1981, 43, 359.
4. D. Chaleil, F. Lefevre, P. Allain and G.J. Martin, J. Inorg. Biochem., 1981, 15, 213.
5. S.B. Coghill, D. Hopwood, S. McPherson and S. Hislop, J. Pathol., 1983, 139, 105.

6. D. Stiel, D.J. Murray and T.J. Peters, Gut, 1985, 26, 364.
7. G.B. van der Voet and F.A. de Wolff, Arch. Toxicol., 1984, 55, 168.
8. D.R. Williams, J. Inorg. Nucl. Chem., 1977, 39, 711.

Transfer of Lead via Rat Milk and Tissue Uptake in the Suckling Offspring

I. Palminger and A. Oskarsson

TOXICOLOGY LABORATORY, NATIONAL FOOD ADMINISTRATION, S-751 26 UPPSALA, SWEDEN

1 INTRODUCTION

The developing nervous system is susceptible to adverse effects of lead. Prenatal exposure and exposure during infancy have been connected with central nervous system dysfunctions including intellectual impairment and behavioural disorders.[1,2] Transfer of lead via milk has been demonstrated in experimental animals,[3] and encephalomyelopathy can easily be induced in suckling rats by adding lead into the diet of lactating dams.[4] There is also metabolic evidence suggesting that the newborn is sensitive to lead. Thus, it has been reported that gastrointestinal absorption and retention of lead are much higher in neonates than in adults, both in humans[5] and in animals.[6]

Although it has been established that lead is transferred into milk in lactating rats, the information is still limited concerning the toxicokinetics of lead during the lactational and immediate postnatal periods. In this study, the transfer of lead into the milk of rats exposed to different doses of lead was examined, as well as the dose-related uptake in the offspring, exposed to lead only through dam's milk.

2 MATERIAL AND METHODS

<u>Animals</u>

Sprague Dawley rats with litters were obtained 10 days after parturition from Möllegaard, Denmark. The rats were individually housed, and provided with R3 pellets (Astra Ewos, Sweden) and tap water *ad libitum*. At the time of arrival, they were randomly divided into six groups of 3-5 rats with litters per group, and the size of each litter was reduced to eight pups.

Experimental Design

On day 15 of lactation the dams were given a single oral dose of ^{203}Pb, specific activity 33 Ci/mmol Pb, purchased from The Svedberg Laboratory, Uppsala University, Sweden. The isotope was either given as such or supplemented with lead acetate in five different doses and administered to the rats by gavage after five h of starvation. The doses were as follows:

Group I: 0.0008 mg (151 µCi) Pb/kg body weight (bw)
Group II: 0.07 mg (283 µCi) Pb/kg bw
Group III: 1.1 mg (141 µCi) Pb/kg bw
Group IV: 6.0 mg (424 µCi) Pb/kg bw
Group V: 10 mg (502 µCi) Pb/kg bw
Group VI: 25 mg (606 µCi) Pb/kg bw

Milk and blood samples were obtained from the dams 24 and 72 h after the administration. At 72 h, all dams were sacrificed after sample collection. The pups were sacrificed 5 h prior to the dams. Liver, brain and kidneys were obtained from all dams and from 3 pups in each litter. Blood was collected from all pups. The radioactivity of ^{203}Pb in milk, blood and tissues was determined in a gamma counter (Nuclear Chicago, Model 4230), using the characteristic line of 279 keV photon emission with a counting efficiency of 47%.

Blood and milk collection.

The pups were separated from the dams five h before milking to allow milk to accumulate in the glands. The dams were anaesthetized with an ip injection of 40 mg/kg bw of sodium pentobarbital (Mebumal vet. ACO, Sweden) followed by a subcutaneous injection of 6.25 U/kg bw of oxytocin (Syntocinon, 5 IE/mL Sandoz, Basel, Switzerland) a few minutes before milking to cause milk let-down. From each dam, 0.5-1 mL milk was obtained by milking several glands with a milking device operated by vacuum, as previously described.[7] Blood was collected by orbital puncture from the dams and by heart puncture from the pups using heparinized capillary tubes and syringes, respectively. To all blood samples, 35 µL of heparin (25000 IU/mL, Kabi Vitrum, Sweden, diluted 1:100) was added. After centrifugation of the blood at 1800 rpm for 15 min, radioactivity was determined in plasma and erythrocytes.

3 RESULTS AND DISCUSSION

The concentration of lead in milk ranged from 0.03 - 131 µg Pb/L and the corresponding blood levels ranged from 0.07 - 109 µg Pb/L 24 h after the administration. The relationship between lead concentrations in the dams' whole blood and milk is shown in Fig. 1A. Linear

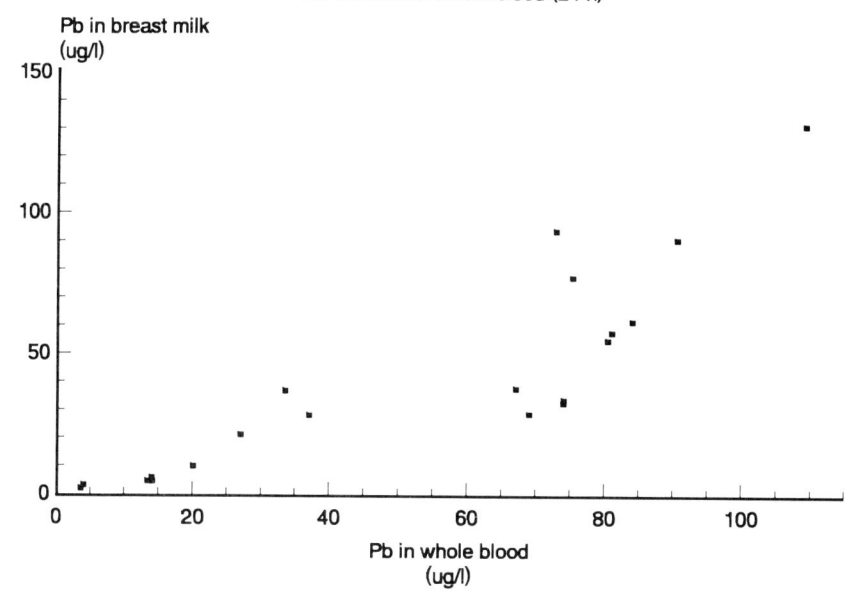

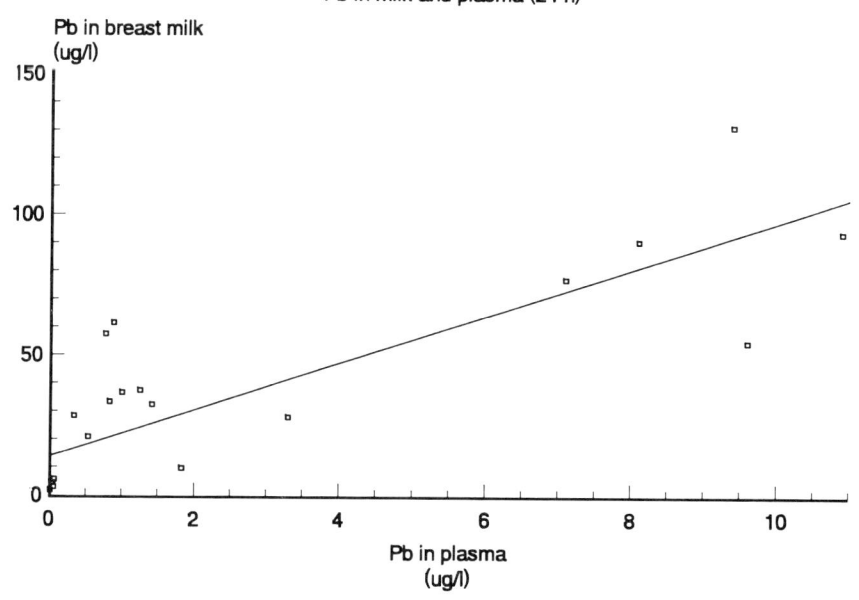

Fig 1. Relationship between lead concentration in whole blood and milk (top) and plasma and milk (bottom) in dams 24 h after a single oral dose of 0.0008-25 mg Pb/kg bw on day 15 of lactation. The regression line $y = 8.9 x + 0.94$ for lead in plasma shows a significant correlation; $r = 0.83$, $p<0.001$.

regression analysis of the data gives a significant correlation, expressed by the equation y (lead in milk) = 0.88 x (lead in whole blood) - 0.48; r = 0.88, p<0.001. This relationship indicates that the level in milk is approx. 80% of the level in whole blood 24 h after the administration. After 72 h, the concentration of lead in milk had decreased by approx 85%, and the ratio between lead in milk and blood had decreased to about 0.3 (y = 0.27 x + 0.07; r = 0.75, p<0.001). The relationship between the levels of lead in blood and milk could also be considered as curvilinear, with the levels in milk becoming progressively greater as the blood lead levels increased. Correlation analysis of the data by best fit polynomial regression gives the equation y = 0.331 + 0.0043 x + 0.95 x^2; r = 0.91. The curvilinear relationship means that the milk/blood ratio decreases with decreasing blood levels of lead. Keller and Doherty found that the milk/blood ratio decreased with time, and consequently also with blood lead levels after a single intravenous or oral dose of lead to lactating mice.[8] Also the plasma/blood ratio decreased with time. However, the milk/plasma ratio was found to be nearly constant in mice over time, and Keller and Doherty[8] concluded that plasma is a more accurate index for the estimation of milk lead concentration than the lead concentration in whole blood.

A linear relationship between the concentration of lead in plasma and milk 24 h after a single oral dose of lead is shown in Fig 1B. The relationship indicates a milk/plasma ratio of eight, which can be compared with a ratio of 25 reported for mice.[8] A similar high milk/plasma ratio was also observed for calcium, and it has been suggested that a common mechanism is involved in the transfer of lead and calcium into milk.[8] The high ratio between lead in milk and plasma is in clear contrast to the low milk/plasma ratios of 0.02-0.2 reported for cadmium,[9] mercury[10] and nickel.[11]

Lead levels in the milk could be used as an indicator of the continuously administered dose of lead to the pups. A significant correlation between lead levels in the milk and in the tissues of the pups was found in this study both at 24 and 72 h after administration. Figures 2A-C show the relationship between the lead concentration in the dams' milk 24 h after the administration, and the brain, liver and kidneys of the pups.

The lead levels in the pups' tissues reached almost the same levels as in the corresponding tissues of the dams, except in the kidneys, where the concentration was much higher in the dams (Table 1). The most striking result is the high concentration of lead in the brain of the sucklings, which might be due to a higher permeability of the blood brain barrier in the immature brain. The low concentration in the kidney of the pups

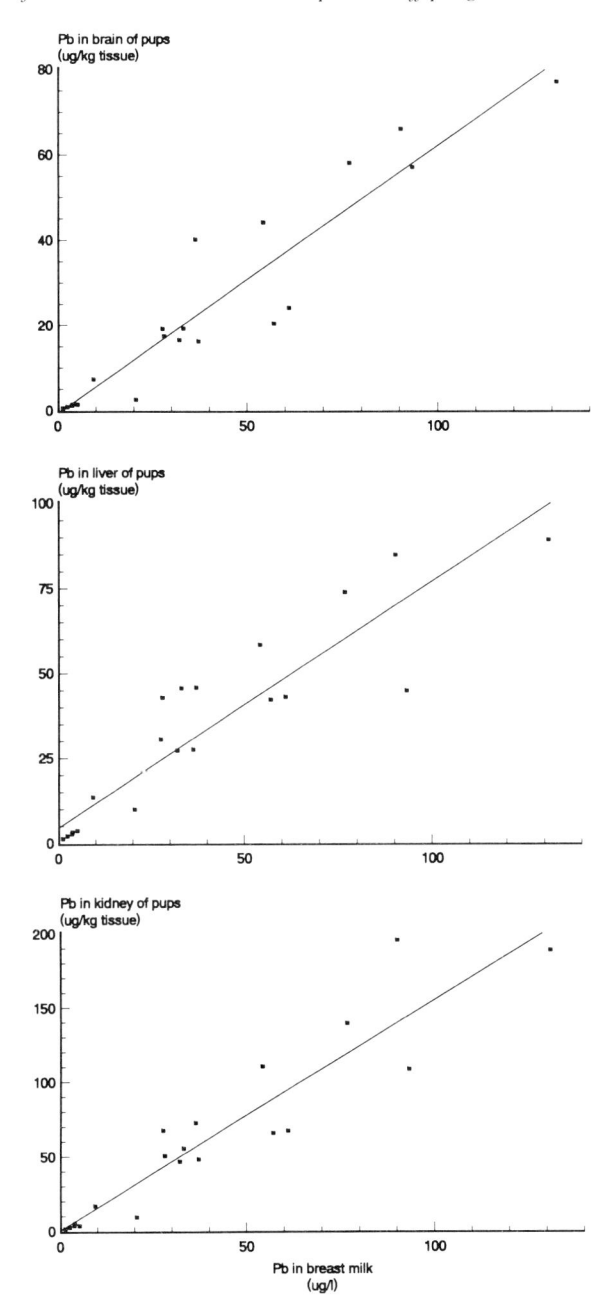

Fig 2. Relationships between lead levels in dams' milk and in brain (top), liver (middle) and kidney (bottom) of the pups which were exposed only through dam's milk. The dams were treated as described in Fig. 1. The regression lines have the equations $y = 0.06 x - 0.07$; $r = 0.95$, $p<0.001$, (brain), $y = 0.73 x + 4.0$; $r = 0.93$, $p<0.001$ (liver), and $y = 1.5 x + 0.17$; $r = 0.95$, $p<0.001$ (kidney).

compared to the dams could be explained by a lower excretory function of the kidneys at this age. A higher absorption and retention in the newborn has also been shown in other studies.[12,13] An important factor of the increased lead absorption in the sucklings could be the milk diet. Kello and Kostial found that the absorption of lead increased in adult rats which received milk together with the normal diet compared to rats which received tap water with the diet.[14]

Table 1. Lead concentration in tissues of dams and pups 72 h after the administration of a single oral dose of lead acetate on day 15 of lactation to the dams. Mean (SEM) values are expressed as ng/g tissue wet weight; n = 3-5 dams and 9-15 pups.

	Dose of lead mg/kg bw				
	0.07	1.1	6.0	10	25
DAMS					
Brain	0.24 (0.03)	2.2 (0.6)	2.1 (0.5)	6.1 (1.4)	8.8 (2.3)
Liver	4.5 (0.9)	40.8 (13)	45.5 (14)	63.3 (18)	82.2 (29)
PUPS					
Brain	0.09 (0.02)	1.4 (0.39)	1.7 (0.35)	4.7 (1)	5.8 (1)
Liver	2.4 (0.4)	31.1 (8.2)	36.0 (7.5)	61.6 (11.5)	53.6 (18.5)
Kidney	2.9 (0.6)	42.0 (11.5)	47.0 (10.5)	128 (26.8)	123 (34)

Human studies have shown lead levels in "unpolluted" milk of about 0.003 mg/kg.[15-17] Higher values of about 0.02 mg/kg have also been reported by Moore and coworkers, and Ryu and coworkers.[18,19] A significant correlation of lead in whole blood and in milk was shown by Moore et al, with the levels in milk being approx. 10% of the levels in blood.[18] Thus, there seems to be a great difference in the transfer of lead into milk in humans from that in rats and mice. Species differences in the binding of lead to erythrocytes, as well as in the milk/plasma ratios of lead, may explain the variations.

4 ACKNOWLEDGEMENT

This study was supported by a grant from the National(Swedish) Environment Protection Board, Project Environmental Health Monitoring System Based on Biological Indicators.

5 REFERENCES

1. J.M. Davis and D.J. Svendsgaard, Nature, 1987, 329, 297.
2. P. Mushak, J.M. Davis, A.F. Crocetti and L.D. Grant, Environ. Res., 1989, 50, 11.
3. R.L. Bornschein, D.A. Fox and I.A. Michaelson, Toxicol. Appl. Pharmacol., 1977, 40, 577.
4. A. Pentschew and F. Garro, Acta Neuropathol., 1966, 6, 266.
5. E.E. Ziegler, B.B. Edwards, R.L. Jensen, K.R. Mahaffey and S.F. Fomon, Pediatr. Res., 1978, 12, 29.
6. K. Kostial, I. Simonovic and M. Pisonic, Nature, 1971, 233, 564.
7. A. Oskarsson, Toxicol. Lett., 1987, 36, 73.
8. C.A. Keller and R.A. Doherty, J. Lab. Clin. Med., 1980, 95, 81.
9. Z. Pietrzak-Flis, G.L. Rehnberg, M.J. Favor, D.F. Cahill and J.W. Laskey, Environ. Res., 1978, 16, 9.
10. F. Bakir, S.F. Damluji, L. Amin-Zaki, M. Murtadha, A. Khalidi, N.Y. Al-Rawi, S. Tikriti, H.I. Dhahir, T.W. Clarkson, J.C. Smith and R.A. Doherty, Science, 1973, 181, 230.
11. L.A. Dostal, S.M. Hopfer, S.-M. Lin and F.W. Sunderman Jr., Toxicol. Appl. Pharmacol., 1989, 101, 220.
12. B. Momcilovic and K. Kostial, Environ. Res., 1974, 8, 214.
13. H.M. Mykkanen, J.W.T. Dickerson and M.C. Lancaster, Toxicol. Appl. Pharmacol., 1979, 51, 447.
14. D. Kello and K. Kostial, Environ. Res., 1973, 6, 355.
15. B. Larsson, S.A. Slorach, U. Hagman and Y. Hofvander, Acta Paediatr. Scand., 1981, 70, 281.
16. S.W. Rockway, C.W. Weber, K.Y. Lei and S.R. Kemberling, Int. Arch. Occup.Environ. Health, 1984, 53, 181.
17. P. Schramel, S. Hasse and J. Ovcar-Pavlu, Biol. Trace Elem. Res., 1988, 15, 111.
18. M.R. Moore, A. Goldberg, S.J. Pocock, A. Meredith, I.M. Stewart, H. MacAnespie, R. Lees and A. Low, Scott. Med. J., 1982, 27, 113.
19. J.E. Ryu, E.E. Ziegler, S.E. Nelson and S.J. Fomon, Am. J. Dis. Child., 1983, 137, 886.

Milk Transfer of Mercury in Rats Given Inorganic or Methylmercury

J. Sundberg and A. Oskarsson

NATIONAL FOOD ADMINISTRATION, TOXICOLOGY LABORATORY, BOX 622, S-751 26 UPPSALA, SWEDEN

1 INTRODUCTION

Exposure to toxic metals during the early neonatal period might cause adverse effects on physical and mental development.[1] However, very little information is available on the toxicokinetics of metals during the lactational and early postnatal period. This period coincides with the period of rapid development of the brain in species such as mouse, rat, dog and man.[2]

Transfer of methylmercury *via* breast milk and uptake in the suckling infant was reported from an outbreak of methylmercury poisoning in Iraq.[3] Two months after the outbreak about 40% of the total mercury in breast milk was in the form of inorganic mercury.[4] In lactating women with a high fish consumption the percentage of inorganic mercury in milk was 80% of the total mercury level.[5] Thus, the suckling infant will be exposed to both inorganic and methylmercury even if the mother is only exposed to methylmercury. There is experimental evidence that inorganic mercury is absorbed more efficiently in suckling animals than in adults.[6] In addition, the excretion of both inorganic and methylmercury is much lower in suckling animals than in adults.[7,8]

In the present study lactating rats were given either inorganic (mercuric Hg^{2+}) mercury or methylmercury. The two forms of mercury were compared concerning the transfer of mercury into milk and the uptake in the offspring.

2 MATERIAL AND METHODS

Sprague-Dawley rats with litters were obtained from Möllegaard, Denmark. Upon arrival the litters were reduced to eight pups, and the sucklings were housed in individual cages with their mothers. The dams were divided into nine groups with three to five dams in each group. The dams were fed a standard R3 diet from Ewos AB, Södertälje, Sweden, and given tap water *ad libitum*.

On either of days 8, 9, 10 or 11 of lactation the dams received a single oral dose of ^{203}mercuric acetate, ^{203}HgAc (specific activity 251 Ci/g Hg), or on day 9 of lactation a single oral dose of methyl^{203}mercuric chloride, CH$_3$^{203}HgCl (specific activity 9.85 mCi/g Hg). Both isotopes were purchased from Amersham International, England. The isotopes were supplemented with unlabelled HgAc and CH$_3$HgCl, respectively. HgAc was dissolved in saline and CH$_3$HgCl in 5 mmol/L Na$_2$CO$_3$. The following doses of ^{203}HgAc were given by gavage. Group I: 0.1 mg (191μCi) Hg/kg body weight (bw), group II: 0.4 mg (539 μCi) Hg/kg bw, group III: 0.7 mg (458 μCi) Hg/kg bw, group IV: 1.3 mg (76 μCi) Hg/kg bw, group V: 5.8 mg (750 μCi) Hg/kg bw. The remaining dams were administered CH$_3$^{203}HgCl in the following doses. Group VI: 0.5 mg (2.48 μCi) Hg/kg bw, group VII: 3.3 mg (16.4 μCi) Hg/kg bw, group VIII: 7.8 mg (46.1 μCi) Hg/kg bw, group IX: 9.4 mg (31.6 μCi) Hg/kg bw.

Using a previously described milking device milk was collected 24 and 72 h after the mercury administration.[9] The dams were separated from the litters for 1-2 h before milking to allow milk to accumulate in the mammary glands. The dams were anaesthetized with an ip injection of 40 mg/kg bw of sodium pentobarbital (Mebumal vet., ACO, Sweden). To cause milk let-down, a subcutaneous injection of 6.25 U oxytocin/kg bw (Syntocinon 5 IE/mL, Sandoz, Basel, Switzerland) was given a few minutes before milking. From each dam, 0.5 - 1 mL of milk was obtained. Immediately after each milking 0.5 mL of blood was collected from the orbital plexus in heparinized capillary tubes and 35 μL of heparin (25 000 IU/mL, Kabi Vitrum, Sweden, diluted 1:100) was added to each blood sample.

Dams with litters were sacrificed after the 72 h milking, blood samples were collected and brain, liver, and kidneys were removed from the mothers and from three pups/litter. Two blood samples were obtained from each litter by heart puncture in heparinized syringes by pooling blood from four pups to each blood sample. Cells and plasma were separated by centrifugation at 1800 rpm for 15 min. The milk was separated into skim milk and fat by centrifugation at 2000 rpm for 15 min. Radioactivity in tissues, blood and milk was measured in a gamma counter (Nuclear Chicago, Model 1185, counting efficiency 51%) for the ^{203}HgAc exposed groups. For radioactivity measurement in the CH$_3$HgCl-exposed groups a Nuclear Chicago Model 4230 was used with a counting efficiency of 35%. The characteristic line of 279 keV photon emission was used.

3 RESULTS AND DISCUSSION

After the administration of inorganic mercury, the concentration in milk significantly decreased from 24 h to 72 h, while after the administration of methylmercury, the concentration in milk remained constant (Table 1). The milk/plasma ratios varied from 0.15 to 0.32 for inorganic mercury and from 0.05 to 0.16 for methylmercury.

Table 1. Mercury in milk. Concentration and distribution of mercury in milk and milk/plasma ratio in lactating dams given one dose of inorganic or methylmercury by gavage on day 8, 9, 10 or 11 of lactation. Milk and blood were collected at 24 h and 72 h after the administration. Mean (SEM) is given; n = 3-5 dams.

Dose mg/kg bw	Hg in milk µg/L 24h	72 h	Per cent Hg in skim milk 24 h	72 h	Milk/Plasma ratio 24 h	72 h
INORGANIC MERCURY						
0.1	0.26 (0.03)	0.11 (0.006)	74 (6)	71 (2)	0.15 (0.02)	0.21 (0.01)
0.4	1.29 (0.13)	0.11 (0.07)	75 (2)	68 (2)	0.18 (0.03)	0.24 (0.03)
0.7	4.83 (0.78)	1.95 (0.20)	79 (1)	69 (3)	0.18 (0.005)	ND
1.3	21.0 (3.8)	8.09 (1.26)	80 (3)	74 (3)	0.18 (0.02)	0.30 (0.02)
5.8	59.9 (16.5)	14.3 (2.5)	78 (6)	77 (7)	0.31 (0.11)	0.32 (0.06)
METHYLMERCURY						
0.5	6.11 (0.82)	6.18 (1.21)	49 (1)	48 (1)	0.05 (0.01)	0.11 (0.02)
3.3	51.6 (3.6)	63.8 (9.3)	45 (4)	45 (2)	0.07 (0.004)	0.16 (0.04)
7.8	206 (9)	160 (20)	42 (2)	48 (1)	0.08 (0.03)	0.07 (0.01)
9.4	226 (2?)	168 (20)	46 (3)	44 (4)	0.11 (0.02)	0.09 (0.02)

ND = Not determined.

In rats treated with methylmercury less than 5% of the mercury in whole blood is present in the plasma fraction.[10] However, after administration of inorganic mercury, approx. 50% of the mercury in whole blood is in the plasma fraction.[10] Most probably the mercury transfer into milk is dependent on the mercury level in plasma and thus, the transfer of inorganic mercury would be favoured. However, the absorption from the gastrointestinal tract is almost complete for methylmercury, while few per cent of inorganic mercury is absorbed.[1,11]

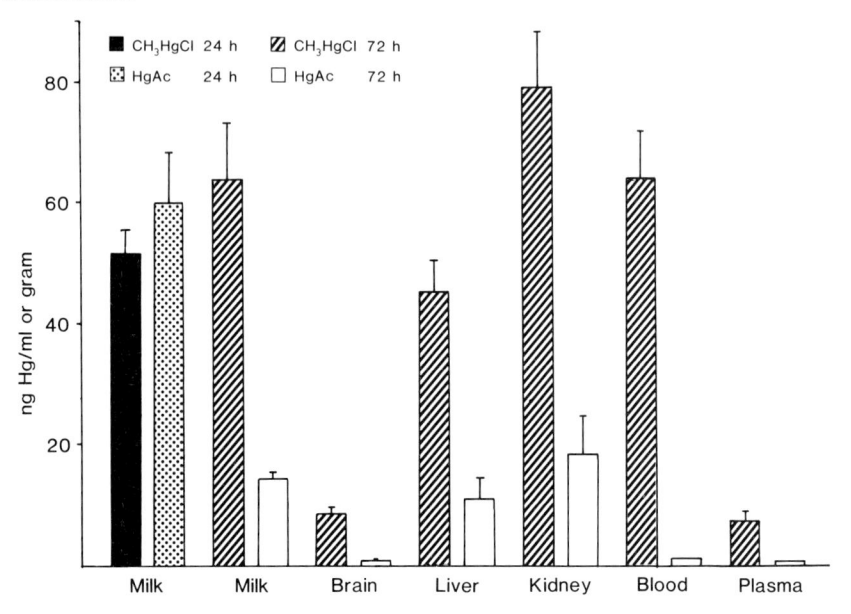

Fig 1. Concentration of mercury in milk from lactating dams at 24 h and 72 h after a single oral dose of 5.8 mg Hg/kg bw of inorganic mercury or 3.3 mg Hg/kg bw of methylmercury on either of days 8 to 11 of lactation and mercury concentration in tissues of their suckling pups at 72 h, expressed as µg/L milk or whole blood or ng Hg/g tissue (wet weight). Mean (SEM) is given; n = 4 dams, 8 pups for blood, 12 pups for tissues.

The distribution of mercury in milk was studied after separating fat from skim milk. There was a higher fraction of mercury in skim milk in the dams treated with inorganic mercury (70-80% in skim milk of the total mercury in milk) compared to dams treated with methylmercury (40-50%) (Table 1). Thus, a significant amount of mercury is found in the fat fraction even after exposure to inorganic mercury (20-30%). Fransson and Lönnerdal studied the distribution of essential metals in milk and found that 15-30% of iron, copper, and zinc in human milk were present in the lipid fraction, predominantly associated to the membrane proteins of the outer fat globule membrane.[12]

The concentration of mercury in milk at 24 h was at a similar level in the two groups given either 5.8 mg/kg bw of inorganic mercury or 3.3 mg/kg bw of methylmercury (Table 1, Fig. 1). The tissue concentrations of mercury were much higher in the sucklings from methylmercury-treated dams than in sucklings from dams treated with inorganic mercury. This can be explained by the continuous high mercury concentration from 24 h to 72 h in the milk of methylmercury-treated dams, as well as by a higher gastrointestinal absorption of methylmercury in the sucklings. Mercury levels in the brain and plasma of sucklings from dams given methylmercury were approximately ten times higher than the corresponding levels in sucklings from dams given inorganic mercury. In whole blood the mercury level was approx. 60 times higher in the former group, suggesting that total mercury level in blood is not a good indicator for the brain level in the newborn. The blood/brain ratio of mercury in the suckling offspring seems to be highly dependent on the chemical form of mercury.

Table 2. Infant/Maternal ratio of mercury. Concentration ratio of mercury in tissues and blood between the offspring and dam, 72 h after the administration of inorganic or methylmercury to dams on either of days 8 to 11 of lactation. Means (SEM) of all dose groups presented in Table 1 (n = 13-19 dams, 26-38 pups for blood, 39-57 pups for tissues) are given.

Tissue	Infant/Maternal Hg-concentration ratio	
	HgAc	CH_3HgCl
Brain	0.030 (0.003)	0.009 (0.0006)
Liver	0.025 (0.002)	0.013 (0.001)
Kidney	0.002 (0.0002)	0.008 (0.0005)
Whole blood	0.010 (0.0008)	0.005 (0.0002)
Erythrocytes	0.010 (0.0007)	0.008 (0.0004)
Plasma	0.019 (0.002)	0.014 (0.002)

The ratios between mercury concentrations in tissues of the offspring and dams are shown in Table 2. The infant/maternal ratios in the groups treated with methylmercury are at a quite constant level, 0.005-0.014, while for inorganic mercury, the ratios range from 0.002 to 0.030. Except for the kidney, there is a higher ratio in the groups treated with inorganic mercury, which was also reported by Mansour et al[13]. They compared the uptake in the offspring of dams given either inorganic or organic mercury subcutaneously 24 h after delivery. After three weeks the infant/maternal ratios were higher than in our study, probably due to the long period of exposure.

The central nervous system is the main target organ for the toxicity of methylmercury.[14] It could be noted that the mercury concentration in the brain in infants is 3% of the maternal concentration in the groups treated with inorganic mercury and only 0.9% in the groups treated with methylmercury. An increasing percentage of the body burden of mercury in the cerebrum was reported by Thomas and Smith,[7] during a two-week long period after a subcutaneous injection of mercuric chloride to 7-day old rats. For inorganic mercury, the main target organ is the kidney.[15] The low renal concentration for sucklings in the inorganic mercury groups in our study, are shown as the low infant/maternal ratio of the kidneys in Table 2. In agreement with our study, other authors have reported a renal/hepatic ratio for inorganic mercury which is lower for sucklings than for adults.[7,13] One explanation is the functional immaturity of the kidneys in the neonate compared to adults.[16]

The results of this study show that the chemical form of mercury is of great importance for the milk transfer and the uptake in the suckling rat. Methylmercury is much more efficiently absorbed from the gastrointestinal tract than inorganic mercury, but the lactational transfer from plasma is greater for inorganic than for methylmercury. The higher infant/maternal ratio of mercury in the group given inorganic mercury may be explained by the fact that inorganic mercury is eliminated from adult rats relatively fast, while the excretion of inorganic mercury in sucklings is delayed.[7]

4   ACKNOWLEDGEMENT

This study was supported by a grant from the National (Swedish) Environment Protection Board, Project Environmental Health Monitoring System based on Biological Indicators.

5   REFERENCES

1. T.W. Clarkson, G.F. Nordberg and P.R. Sager, Scand. J. Work Environ. Health., 1985, 11, 145.
2. A.N. Davison and J. Dobbing, 'Applied Neurochemistry' Blackwell Sci Publications, Oxford and Edinburgh, 1968, p. 253.
3. E. Bakir, S.F. Damluji, L. Amin-Zaki, M. Murtadha, A. Khalidi, N.Y. Al-Rawi, S. Tikriti, H.I. Dhahir, T.W. Clarkson, J.C. Smith and R.A. Doherty, Science, 1973, 181, 230.

4. L. Amin-Zaki, S. Elhassani, M.A. Majeed, T.W. Clarkson, R.A. Doherty, M.R. Greenwood and T. Giovanoli-Jakubszak, Am. J. Dis. Child., 1976, 130, 1070.
5. S. Skerfving, Bull. Environ. Contam. toxicol., 1988, 41, 475.
6. K. Kostial, 'Reproductive and Developmental Toxicity of Metals', T.W. Clarkson, G.F. Nordberg, P.R. Sager, eds, Plenum Press, New York and London, 1983, p.727.
7. D.J. Thomas and J.C. Smith, Toxicol. Appl. Pharmacol., 1979, 48, 43.
8. I.R. Rowland, R.D. Robinson, R.A. Doherty and T.D. Landry, 'Reproductive and Developmental Toxicity of Metals', T.W. Clarkson, G.F. Nordberg, P.R. Sager, eds, Plenum Press, New York and London, 1983, p.745.
9. A. Oskarsson, Toxicol. Lett., 1987, 36, 73.
10. G. F. Nordberg and S. Skerfving, 'Mercury in the Environment', L. Friberg and J. Vostal, eds, CRC Press, Cleveland, Ohio, 1972, 4, p. 29.
11. K. Kostial, D. Kello, S. Jugo, I. Rabar and T. Maljkovic, Environ. Health Persp., 1978, 25, 81.
12. G. Fransson and B. Lönnerdal, Pediatr. Res., 1983, 17, 912.
13. M. M. Mansour, N.C. Dyer, L.H. Hoffman, A.R. Schulert and A.B. Brill, Environ. Res., 1973, 6, 479.
14. IPCS 'Environmental Health Criteria 101. Methylmercury.', World Health Organization, Geneva, 1990.
15. C. E. Ganote, K.A. Reimer and R.B. Jennings, Lab. Invest., 1974, 31, 633.
16. M. Webb and D. Holt, Arch. Toxicol., 1982, 49, 237.

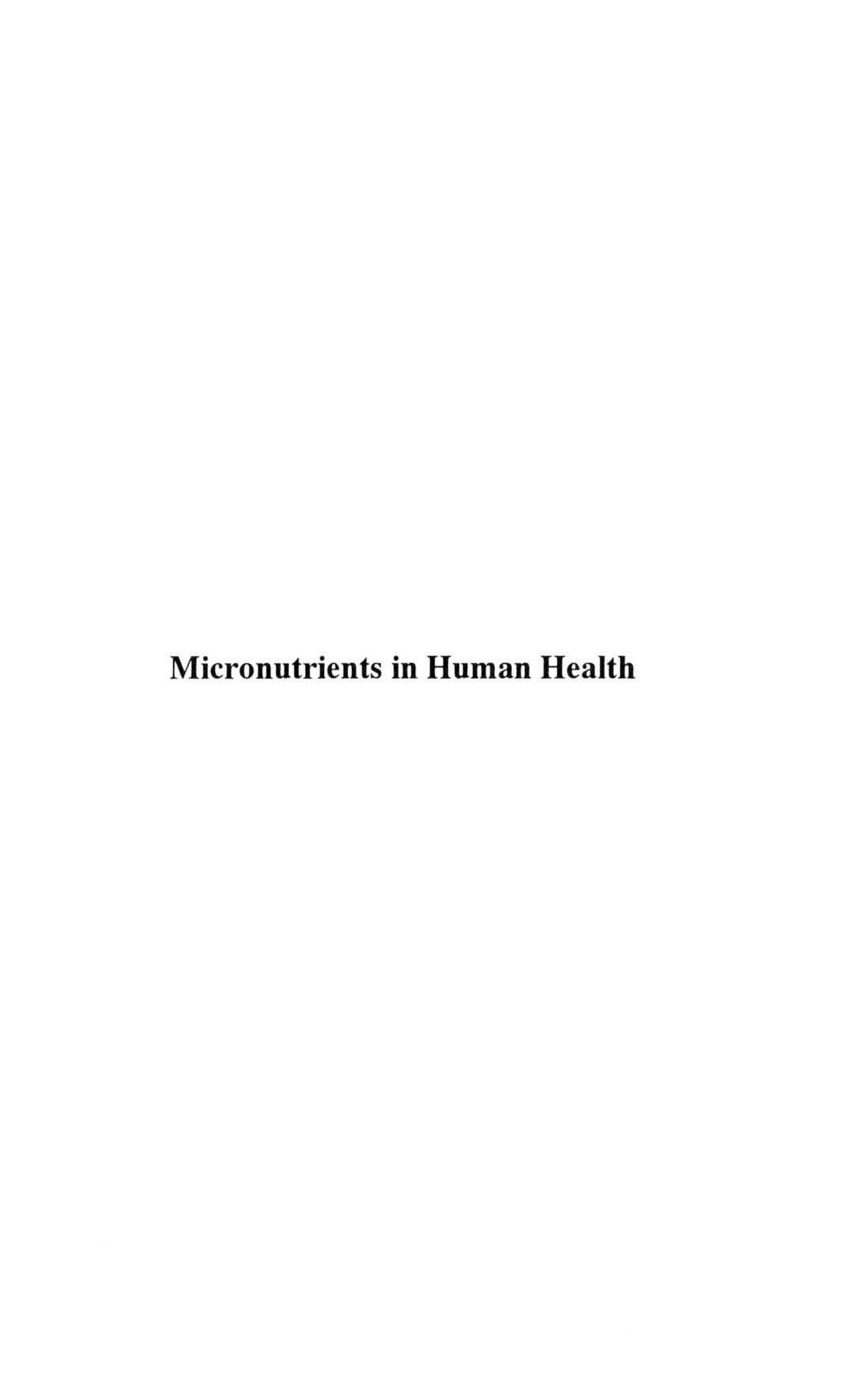

Micronutrients in Human Health

Micronutrients and Cardiovascular Disease

J. Virtamo and J. K. Huttunen

NATIONAL PUBLIC HEALTH INSTITUTE, MANNERHEIMINTIE 166, SF-00300 HELSINKI, FINLAND

1 INTRODUCTION

Several factors have been found to be associated with an increased risk of major manifestations of atherosclerotic disease in man[1]. The most common are abnormalities in hemostatic functions, lipids and lipoproteins, and elevated blood pressure and cigarette smoking. Many of these factors are influenced by diet, and thus the association between diet and cardiovascular disease has been intensively studied during the past decades.

Improved analytical methods and rapidly expanding knowledge of the physiological functions of micronutrients have attracted increasing attention to the role of these substances in the etiology of human diseases. This review summarizes current knowledge on the relationship between cardiovascular diseases and trace elements and vitamins.

2 TRACE ELEMENTS

Chromium

There is some evidence that chromium has a role in the pathogenesis of cardiovascular disease in experimental animals. Schroeder[2] reported that chromium deficiency leads to elevation of serum cholesterol and to formation of aortic plaques in rat. These changes were reversed by chromium supplementation. Regression of cholesterol-induced aortic plaques during chromium feeding has also been described in rabbits[3].

Data on the association between chromium and the risk of cardiovascular disease in man are scarce and conflicting. Subjects dying of ischemic heart disease had lower aortic chromium concentrations than did those dying of accidents or other diseases[4]. In one study[5] patients with angiographically proven coronary heart disease had lower serum chromium concentrations than subjects with normal coronary arteries, while no differences were observed in another study[6] of similar design. The urinary chromium excretion of subjects with definite atherosclerotic disease did not differ from that of healthy controls[7]. Investigations relating the chromium content of drinking water to the risk of cardiovascular disease have produced contradictory results[8-14]. The evaluation of all these studies is complicated by the fact that inadequate analytical methods for measuring chromium have been in use[15].

The effects of chromium on glucose metabolism have been studied extensively in both animals and man since the initial suggestion that a chromium compound in brewer's yeast influences glucose control[16]. However, recent experimental studies have not confirmed earlier findings suggesting that chromium supplementation improves glucose tolerance in chromium-deficient rats[17]. The data on the effect of chromium on glucose tolerance in man is also conflicting. Supplemental chromium has been reported to improve glucose tolerance in patients sustained on total parenteral nutrition[18]. On the other hand, chromium supplementation has not generally influenced blood glucose levels in subjects with overt diabetes[19-21]. Nevertheless, subjects with milder forms of glucose intolerance may respond to chromium feeding. Thus, an improvement of glucose control after chromium supplementation has been reported in elderly people[22-25] and in middle-aged subjects with mild glucose intolerance and/or hyperinsulinemia[26-28].

It has been suggested that chromium influences the number or affinity of insulin receptors in peripheral tissues[27,29]. In agreement with this hypothesis chromium supplementation has in some studies lowered the response of plasma insulin to glucose loads[20,23,26]. These findings are interesting as hyperinsulinemia is possibly an important risk factor of coronary disease in man[30,31].

Reports of the effects of chromium on serum lipids in man are controversial. A fall in total serum cholesterol and/or a rise in HDL cholesterol has been observed in some studies[23,26,28,32]. However, most controlled studies have failed to demonstrate consistent changes in lipid or lipoprotein concentrations after chromium supplementation[19-21,27,33,34].

Interpretation of the data on the effects of chromium on lipid and glucose metabolism is difficult for several reasons[15]. Firstly, a reliable laboratory marker to diagnose chromium deficiency is missing. Thus, it is not possible to screen for subjects who have simultaneous chromium deficiency and abnormalities in glucose or lipid metabolism, and so subjects with these disorders as well as those with normal chromium status are included in supplementation trials. Secondly, the organic compound assumed to be the biologically active form of chromium[16] has not yet been characterized and is thus not available for supplementation studies. In investigations using inorganic chromium, differences in absorption and/or conversion to the hypothetical active form may have obscured the effects on glucose and lipid metabolism.

Selenium

Selenium deficiency is associated with cardiomyopathy and sudden death, both in experimental and domestic animals. Severe selenium deficiency is also involved in the pathogenesis of cardiomyopathy in man. Studies conducted in the People's Republic of China have shown that Keshan disease, a cardiomyopathy mainly affecting children and women of child-bearing age, can be prevented by supplementation with sodium selenite[35]. Keshan disease closely resembles the cardiomyopathy seen in selenium-deficient animals; the characteristic finding is focal myocardial necrosis without changes in coronary arteries. The disease is fatal in a high percentage of cases. Selenium deficiency alone may not precipitate the clinical disease. It has been speculated that another factor, either a viral infection or high dietary intake of erucic acid-containing fats, is needed for symptomatic disease[36,37].

Congestive cardiomyopathy with low selenium levels has also been reported in patients receiving total parenteral nutrition[38,39]. Fatal cases have been characterized by widespread myocytolysis and fibrosis, features resembling those observed in Keshan disease and the cardiomyopathy of selenium-deficient animals[38].

Selenium is a constituent of glutathione peroxidase, an enzyme with an important function in eliminating hydrogen peroxide and organic hydroperoxides[40]. Low glutathione peroxidase activity may lead to accumulation of fatty acid hydroperoxides, thereby inhibiting the synthesis of prostacyclin in the blood vessel wall and tipping the thromboxane-prostacyclin balance toward the proaggregatory state[41]. Indeed, decreased prostacyclin production in the aorta and increased platelet aggregation have been reported in rats after selenium depletion[42-44]. Furthermore, platelets from selenium-deficient rats produce more thromboxane when stimulated by ADP and collagen than do platelets from normal rats[44]. Lipid hydroperoxides may also cause direct injury to the vessel endothelium.

An association between selenium deficiency and coronary heart disease in man was originally suggested on the basis of regional comparisons of coronary heart disease rates and dietary selenium intakes[45]. The results of studies in patients with coronary disease have been less consistent. While some investigators have found a reduced serum selenium level in subjects with myocardial infarction or angiographically verified coronary disease[46,47], others have not[6,48]. Kok et al.[49] reported a lower toenail selenium level in patients with acute myocardial infarction than in healthy controls. This observation is important as it suggests that dietary intake of selenium had been low in patients during the months preceding infarction.

The prospective follow-up studies on the association between serum selenium and the risk of coronary heart disease have shown varying results. It appears that a dietary intake of selenium maintaining serum selenium above 45 µg/L does not contribute to the development of ischemic heart disease. The association between coronary risk and a serum selenium level below 45 µg/L is uncertain, since one study demonstrated a significant association[50], two studies showed a weak or no association[51,52], and other prospective studies have not included subjects with serum selenium concentrations below 45 µg/L[53-56].

Preliminary observations also suggest that selenium influences platelet aggregability in man. Selenium inhibited the production of thromboxane A_2 in platelets, but had no effect on endothelial prostacyclin synthesis in vitro[57]. Furthermore, a recent study demonstrated an inverse association between serum selenium and platelet aggregability in men with coronary heart disease[58]. These findings might explain the increased risk of stroke and coronary death in subjects with low serum selenium, observed in prospective follow-up studies[50,51].

Zinc

A diet containing several times more zinc than required for normal growth reduced the incidence and severity of aortic and cerebral atherosclerosis in rats[59]. In one study human subjects with hyperlipoproteinemia and symptoms of atherosclerosis had lower serum zinc concentrations than hyperlipoproteinemic subjects without symptoms[60]. In contrast, serum zinc levels were similar in subjects with angiographically verified coronary heart disease and in subjects with normal coronary arteries[6]. A third study found no difference in baseline serum zinc concentration between survivors and men dying of coronary disease in a ten-year prospective study[61].

Experiments by Klevay and his associates in rats have suggested that a high dietary ratio of zinc to copper raises serum cholesterol level[62], but these findings have not been replicated by other investigators[63-67]. The findings in man are divergent. A high dose of zinc (160 mg daily) lowered HDL-cholesterol but did not influence total cholesterol in the study reported by Hooper et al.[68]. A slightly lower dose of zinc (100 mg daily) induced a transient decrease in HDL cholesterol after four weeks[69]. More physiological doses of zinc have had no effect on total and HDL cholesterol[69-71].

Diabetics often have an increased urinary excretion of zinc and an abnormally low serum zinc concentration[72,74], and it has been suggested that zinc deficiency might play a role in impaired T-cell function and in the pathogenesis of diabetic foot ulcers[75]. However, zinc supplementation did not influence the level of glycosylated hemoglobin in subjects with Type II diabetes[74]. Acute zinc depletion has been reported to impair platelet aggregation and to decrease the sensitivity to aggregating agents both in man and in experimental animals[76].

Copper

Severe copper deficiency is associated with cardiovascular abnormalities in several animal species. Aortic lesions observed in experimental animals are assumed to be caused by impaired function of lysyl oxidase, a copper-containing enzyme essential for the structural integrity of vascular connective tissue[77]. The characteristic findings seen in the myocardium include hypertrophy with hemorrhage, inflammation and focal necrosis, but no changes in coronary arteries[59,77].

Severe copper deficiency raises serum cholesterol in rats and mice[77-79], while copper intakes corresponding to the amounts present in normal western diets do not influence plasma lipid levels in animals[63,64]. Other metabolic abnormalities described in copper-deficient animals include glucose intolerance[80-82] and hyperuricemia[83]. On the other hand, severe copper deficiency has consistently been associated with lowered blood pressure in rats[84-86].

Copper is found at the active site of the superoxide dismutase enzyme which deactivates the superoxide radical. Thus, a marginal copper status could promote atherosclerosis via oxidative damage caused by reduced activity of this enzyme. However, an increased mean serum copper concentration was observed among men with angiographically verified coronary heart disease[6]. In a longitudinal study, the adjusted risk of death from cardiovascular disease was about four times higher for subjects in the highest serum copper quintile as compared to those with normal levels[87]. The high serum copper levels seen in subjects with atherosclerotic heart disease could, however, be a result rather than the cause of the disease as ceruloplasmin, the main carrier of copper in serum, is elevated in various acute and chronic diseases[88]. On the other hand, an increased risk was also observed in subjects in the lowest serum copper quintile, suggesting that the association is U-shaped[87].

The effect of copper on blood lipids in humans is not well defined. A positive correlation has been described in cross-sectional studies between serum copper and total serum cholesterol concentration[6,89], whereas an inverse association has been found between serum copper and HDL cholesterol[89]. In a depletion-repletion study with 24 males, an experimental diet inadequate in copper (0.36 mg per day per 1000 kcal) for 11 weeks induced significant increases in LDL cholesterol and significant decreases in HDL cholesterol when compared to a repletion diet (1.41 mg copper per day per 1000 kcal)[90].

Other Trace Elements

Magnesium deficiency induces cardiac arrhythmias both in experimental animals and humans[91,92]. A transient hypomagnesemia is a common finding in patients with acute myocardial infarction[92-94]. There is evidence that administration of intravenous magnesium prevents hypomagnesemia, diminishes the size of myocardial infarction and results in lower mortality rates in patients with acute myocardial infarction[95-98]. Some studies suggest that magnesium might also be involved in the pathogenesis of atherosclerotic disease, but the evidence is so far not convincing[99,100].

Ecological comparisons have provided some evidence that populations living in areas with a low fluoride content of drinking water have increased cardiovascular morbidity[13,101,102]. These studies are contrasted by other investigations which have found no relationship between regional cardiovascular mortality and fluoride in drinking water[103-106]. A significant inverse association between the risk of myocardial infarction and the fluoride concentration in drinking water was found in a case-control study from Finland[107]. There is no data on the effects of low or high fluoride intakes on serum lipids, blood pressure or other risk factors of cardiovascular disease.

3 VITAMINS

Vitamin A and Beta-carotene

Information on the association between cardiovascular disease and vitamin A and its precursor, beta-carotene, is very limited. Serum retinol concentration did not predict cardiovascular mortality in two follow-up studies[52,55]. No significant effects of administration of beta-carotene on any of the major cardiovascular end points were observed during the first 60 months in a controlled trial with over 22 000 American physicians[108].

Vitamin E

The effects of vitamin E on intermittent claudication have been examined in dozens of trials. Some have suggested the usefulness of vitamin E in long-term treatment programmes, while others have failed to detect any changes in clinical symptoms[109]. In Haeger's open trial[110] some improvement in walking distance was observed after 3-4 months of treatment, although objective changes in the arterial circulation were only detectable after 18 months. The interpretation of all these observations is rendered difficult by the fact that intermittent claudication is characterized by fluctuating severity of symptoms, and some cases improve without any treatment. A large, long-term double-blind trial would obviously be needed to confirm or refute the findings of previous small-scale studies.

A report published in 1946 suggested that high doses of vitamin E would diminish or abolish anginal pain[111]. Since then more than ten investigations, including some double-blind controlled studies, have failed to confirm the finding[109].

Some observations suggest that vitamin E status might influence the risk of atherosclerotic disease in man. Gey et al.[112] found that serum tocopherol levels were lower in 40-49-year old men from countries with high incidences of coronary heart disease (Finland, Scotland) than in men from lands with low incidence (Italy, Switzerland). An ecological study based on the WHO MONICA populations showed a relatively strong correlation between coronary mortality and serum alpha-tocopherol corrected for serum cholesterol levels[113]. On the other hand, follow-up studies within populations have failed to establish an association between serum alpha-tocopherol levels and cardiovascular mortality[52,55,112].

Vitamin E has several effects on the cardiovascular system that could be involved in the pathogenesis of coronary heart disease and stroke. Vitamin E deficiency reduces prostacyclin production in experimental animals, and these changes are reversed by vitamin E supplementation[114]. In vitro studies of human blood platelets have shown that vitamin E lowers thromboxane A_2 production[57] and inhibits platelet aggregation[115]. In vivo studies in healthy volunteers have not generally shown an effect on platelet aggregation[116,117]. Diabetes is associated with platelet aggregation disturbances and abnormal prostaglandin production, both of which may respond favourably to vitamin E[118]. Vitamin E may also weaken the clotting activity of platelets caused by the use of contraceptive pills[119].

Large doses of vitamin E may exacerbate coagulation defects due to vitamin K deficiency caused by malabsorption syndromes, diet, or the administration of anticoagulant drugs[120]. The mechanism of this interaction is not known. In healthy volunteers, vitamin E does not influence the coagulation process.

There has been much research into the significance of vitamin E on blood lipids. Herman et al.[121] published findings suggesting that vitamin E supplementation raises HDL cholesterol. Subsequent studies have not been able to substantiate this observation, although there have been occasional reports of a beneficial effect of the vitamin E on HDL cholesterol, when initial levels of HDL cholesterol were low or total cholesterol high (for a review, see ref. 120). Vitamin E has no effect on serum total cholesterol or triglycerides.

Attention has recently been focused on oxidative modification of LDL, a process which might enhance the atherogenicity of this lipoprotein[122]. In kinetics study with human LDL no formation of oxidatively modified LDL was detectable until all of the endogenous alpha-tocopherol of LDL had been consumed[123]. Similarly, in vivo supplementation of alpha-tocopherol extended the duration of the lag period during which no detectable oxidative modification of LDL occurred. Treatment of diabetic rats with vitamin E has been shown to inhibit *in vivo* oxidation and in vitro cytotoxicity of LDL and VLDL[124,125]. Whether vitamin E also protects against atherosclerosis by preventing oxidation of LDL remains to be shown.

Vitamin C

Epidemiological evidence for a link between vitamin C intake and ischemic heart disease is weak. In a five-country comparison Gey et al.[112] found that 40-49-year old men in the countries with the highest and medium coronary mortalities (N.Ireland, Scotland and Finland) had lower serum vitamin C levels than men of similar age in Italy and Switzerland, where coronary heart disease rates are lower. In the only follow-up study published so far, there was no difference in serum vitamin C levels between men dying from ischemic heart disease and the survivors[112].

In experimental animals, vitamin C deficiency raises blood cholesterol levels and promotes atherosclerosis[126]. These changes are reversed by ascorbic acid supplements. Early uncontrolled investigations suggested that vitamin C has a similar effect in man. However, placebo-controlled experiments have consistently shown lack of effect in subjects with normal or marginally adequate intakes of vitamin C[127-130].

Vitamin C has been reported to influence prostaglandin metabolism. Toivanen[57] found that in vitro vitamin C almost doubled human endothelial cell prostacyclin output, while the concurrent blood platelet thromboxane A_2 production remained essentially unchanged.

4 REFERENCES

1. J. Stamler,"Nutrition, Lipids, and Coronary Heart Disease: a Global View", R. Levy, B. Rifkind, B. Dennis, N. Ernst, eds., Raven Press, New York, 1979, p. 25.
2. H.A. Schroeder, Am.J.Clin.Nutr., 1968, 21, 230.
3. A.S. Abraham, M. Sonnenblick and M. Eini, Atherosclerosis, 1982, 42, 185.
4. H.A. Schroeder, A.P. Nason and I.H. Tipton, J.Chron.Dis., 1970, 23, 123.
5. H.A.I. Newman, R.F. Leighton, R.R. Lanese and N.A. Freedland, Clin.Chem., 1978, 24, 541.
6. J. Manthey, M. Stoeppler, W. Morgenstern, E. Nüssel, D. Opherk, A. Weintraut, H. Wesch and W. Kübler, Circulation, 1981, 64, 722.
7. S. Punsar, W. Wolf, W. Mertz and M.J. Karvonen, Ann.Clin.Res., 1977, 9, 79.
8. S. Punsar, O. Erämetsä, M.J. Karvonen, A. Ryhänen, P. Hilska and H. Vornamo, J.Chron.Dis., 1975, 28, 259.
9. S. Punsar and M.J. Karvonen, Cardiology, 1979, 64, 24.
10. R. Masironi, Bull. WHO, 1970, 43, 687.
11. A.W. Voors, Am.J.Epidemiol., 1971, 93, 259.
12. H.A. Schroeder, JAMA, 1966, 195, 125.
13. M.D. Crawford, M.J. Gardner and J.N. Morris, Lancet, 1968, i, 827.
14. H.I. Sauer, D.W. Parke and M.L. Neill, "Trace Substances in Environmental Health", D.D. Hemphill, ed., University of Missouri, Columbia, Missouri, 1971, p. 318.
15. E.G. Offenbacher and F.X. Pi-Sunyer, Ann.Rev.Nutr., 1988, 8, 543.
16. W. Mertz, Nutr.Rev., 1975, 33, 129.
17. D.L. Donaldson, D.M. Lee, C.C. Smith and O.M. Rennert, Metabolism, 1985, 34, 1086.
18. H. Freund, S. Atamian and J.E. Fischer, JAMA, 1979, 241, 496.
19. M.B. Rabinowitz, H.C. Gonick, S.R. Levin and M.B. Davidson, Diabetes Care, 1983, 6, 319.
20. M.I.J. Uusitupa, J.T. Kumpulainen, E. Voutilainen, K. Hersio, H. Sarlund, K.P. Pyörälä, P.E. Koivistoinen and J.T. Lehto, Am.J.Clin.Nutr., 1983, 38, 404.
21. A.E. Hunt, K.G.D. Allen and B.A. Smith, Nutr.Res., 1985, 5, 131.
22. R.A. Levine, D.H.P. Streeten and R.J. Doisy, Metabolism, 1968, 17, 114.
23. E.G. Offenbacher and F.X. Pi-Sunyer, Diabetes, 1980, 29, 919.

24. J.F. Potter, P. Levin, R.A. Anderson, J.M. Freiberg, R. Andres and D. Elahi, Metabolism, 1985, 34, 199.
25. M. Urberg and M.B. Zemel, Metabolism, 1987, 36, 896.
26. R. Riales and M.J. Albrink, Am.J.Clin.Nutr., 1981, 34, 2670.
27. R.A. Anderson, M.M. Polansky, N.A. Bryden, E.E. Roginski, W. Mertz and W. Glinsmann, Metabolism, 1983, 32, 894.
28. J.A. Vinson and P. Bose, Nutr.Rep.Int., 1984, 30, 911.
29. K.M. Hambidge, Am.J.Clin.Nutr., 1974, 27, 505.
30. K. Pyörälä, Diabetes Care, 1979, 2, 131.
31. G.M. Reaven and B.B. Hoffman, Am.J.Med., 1989, 87, Suppl. 6A, 2.
32. J.C. Elwood, D.T. Nash and D.H.P. Streeten, J.Am.Coll.Nutr., 1982, 1, 263.
33. E.G. Offenbacher, C.J. Rinko and F.X. Pi-Sunyer, Am.J.Clin.Nutr., 1985, 42, 454.
34. D.M. Bourn, R.S. Gibson, O.B. Martinez and A.C. MacDonald, Biol.Trace Element Res., 1986, 9, 197.
35. X. Chen, G. Yang, J. Chen, X. Chen, Z. Wen and K. Ge, Biol.Trace Element Res., 1980, 2, 91.
36. M. Wen, Y.S. Chen, P. Fu, C.H. Quian, W.R. Liu and H.J. Huang, "Selenium in Biology and Medicine", G.F. Combs Jr., J.E. Spallholz, O.A. Levander and J.E. Oldfield, eds., Van Nostrand Reinhold, New York, 1987, Part B, p. 902.
37. M.D. Laryea, Y.F. Jiang, G.L. Xu, D. Frosch and I. Lombeck, "Selenium in Biology and Medicine", A. Wendel, ed., Springer-Verlag, Berlin, 1989, p. 277.
38. R.A. Johnson, S.S. Baker, J.T. Fallon, E.P. Maynard, J.N. Ruskin, Z. Wen, K.Ge and H.J. Cohen, N.Engl.J.Med., 1981, 304, 1210.
39. K. Sriram, J.K. Peterson, J. O'Gara, J.M. Hammond, Acta Pharmacol.Toxicol., 1986, 59, Suppl. 7, 361.
40. G.F. Combs Jr. and S.B. Combs, Annu.Rev.Nutr., 1984, 4, 257.
41. S. Moncada and J.R. Vane, N.Engl.J.Med., 1979, 300, 1142.
42. H. Bult, P. Van den Bosch, R. Van den Bossche, A. Van Hoydonck and A.G. Herman, Thromb.Haemost., 1981, 46, 272.
43. T. Masukawa, J. Goto and H. Iwata, Experientia, 1983, 39, 405.
44. N.W. Schoene, V.C. Morris and O.A. Levander, Nutr.Res., 1986, 6, 75.
45. R.J. Shamberger, "Selenium in Biology and Medicine", J.E. Spallholz, J.L. Martin and H.E. Ganther, eds., AVI Publishing, Westport, Conneticut, 1981, p. 391.
46. O. Oster, M. Drexler, J. Schenk, T. Meinertz, W. Kasper, C.J. Schuster and W. Prellwitz, Ann.Clin.Res., 1986, 18, 36.
47. J.A. Moore, R. Noiva and I.C. Wells, Clin.Chem., 1984, 30, 1171.
48. A. Aro, G. Alfthan, S. Soimakallio and E. Voutilainen, Clin.Chem., 1986, 32, 911.

49. F.J. Kok, A. Hofman, J.C.M. Witteman, A.M. de Bruijn, D.H.C.M. Kruyssen, M. de Bruin and H.A. Valkenburg, JAMA, 1989, 261, 1161.
50. J.T. Salonen, G. Alfthan, J.K. Huttunen, J. Pikkarainen and P. Puska, Lancet, 1982, ii, 175.
51. J. Virtamo, E. Valkeila, G. Alfthan, S. Punsar, J.K. Huttunen and M.J. Karvonen, Am.J.Epidemiol., 1985, 122, 276.
52. J.T. Salonen, R. Salonen, I. Penttilä, J. Herranen, M. Jauhiainen, M. Kantola, R. Lappeteläinen, P.H. Mäenpää, G. Alfthan and P. Puska, Am.J.Cardiol., 1985, 56, 226.
53. T.A. Miettinen, G. Alfthan, J.K. Huttunen, J. Pikkarainen, V. Naukkarinen, S. Mattila and T. Kumlin, Br.Med.J., 1983, 287, 517.
54. J. Ringstad and D. Thelle, Acta Pharmacol.Toxicol., 1986, 59, Suppl. 7, 336.
55. F.J. Kok, A.M. de Bruijn, R. Vermeeren, A. Hofman, A. van Laar, M. de Bruin, R.J.J. Hermus and H.A. Valkenburg, Am.J.Clin.Nutr., 1987, 45, 462.
56. J. Ringstad, B.K. Jacobsen, Y. Thomassen and D.S. Thelle. J.Epidemiol.Community Health, 1987, 41, 329.
57. J.L. Toivanen, Prostaglandins Leukotrienes Med., 1987, 26, 265.
58. J.T. Salonen, R. Salonen, K. Seppänen, M. Kantola, M. Parviainen, G. Alfthan, P.H. Mäenpää, E. Taskinen and R. Rauramaa, Atherosclerosis, 1988, 70, 155.
59. H.G. Petering, L. Murthy, K.L. Stemmer, V.N. Finelli and E.E. Mendcn, Biol.Trace Element Res., 1986, 9, 251.
60. G. Uza, S. Gabor, A. Kovats, R. Vlaicu and M. Cucuianu, Biol.Trace Element Res., 1985, 8, 167.
61. J. Niskanen, J. Marniemi, O. Piironen, J. Maatela, J. Mäki, I. Vuori, A. Seppänen, V. Kallio and A. Aromaa, Acta Pharmacol.Toxicol., 1986, 59, Suppl. 7, 340.
62. L.M. Klevay, Am.J.Clin.Nutr., 1973, 26, 1060.
63. W.O. Caster and J.M. Doster, Nutr.Rep.Int., 1979, 19, 773.
64. P.W.F. Fischer, A. Giroux, B. Belonje and B.G. Shah, Am.J.Clin.Nutr., 1980, 33, 1019.
65. W. Woo, D.L. Gibbs, P.L. Hooper and P.J. Garry, Am.J.Clin.Nutr., 1981, 34, 120.
66. M. Lefevre, C.L. Keen, B. Lönnerdal, L.S. Hurley and B.O. Schneeman, J.Nutr., 1985, 115, 359.
67. N.A. Frimpong and A.C. Magee, Nutr.Rep.Int., 1987, 35, 551.
68. P.L. Hooper, L. Visconti, P.J. Garry and G.E. Johnson, JAMA, 1980, 244, 1960.
69. J.H. Freeland-Graves, B.J. Friedman, W. Han, R.L. Shorey and R. Young, Am.J.Clin.Nutr., 1982, 35, 988.
70. J.H. Freeland-Graves, W. Han, B.J. Friedman and R.L. Shorey. Nutr.Rep.Int., 1980, 22, 285.
71. S.F. Crouse, P.L. Hooper, H.A. Atterbom and R.L. Papenfuss. JAMA, 1984, 252, 785.

72. W.B. Kinlaw, A.S. Levine, J.E. Morley, S.E. Silvis and C.J. McClain, Am.J.Med., 1983, 75, 273.
73. P. McNair, S. Kiilerich, C. Christiansen, M.S. Christensen, S. Madsbad and I. Transbol, Clin.Chim.Acta, 1981, 112, 343.
74. C.B. Niewoehner, J.I. Allen, M. Boosalis, A.S. Levine and J.E. Morley, Am.J.Med., 1986, 81, 63.
75. A.D. Mooradian and J.E. Morley, Am.J.Clin.Nutr., 1987, 45, 877.
76. P.R. Gordon and B.L. O'Dell, J.Nutr., 1983, 113, 239.
77. K.G.D. Allen and L.M. Klevay, Atherosclerosis, 1978, 29, 81.
78. K.G.D. Allen and L.M. Klevay, Atherosclerosis, 1978, 31, 259.
79. K.G.D. Allen and L.M. Klevay, Nutr.Rep.Int., 1980, 22, 295.
80. A.M. Cohen, A. Teitelbaum, E. Miller, V. Ben-Tor, R. Hirt and M. Fields, Isr.J.Med.Sci., 1982, 18, 840.
81. C.A. Hassel, J.A. Marchello and K.Y. Lei, J.Nutr., 1983, 113, 1081.
82. L.M. Klevay, Nutr.Rep.Int., 1982, 26, 329.
83. L.M. Klevay, Nutr.Rep.Int., 1980, 22, 617.
84. M. Fields, R.J. Ferretti, J.C. Smith Jr. and S. Reiser, Life Sci., 1984, 34, 763.
85. D.M. Medeiros, K. Lin, C.F. Liu and B.M. Thorne, Nutr.Rep.Int., 1984, 30, 559.
86. B.N. Wu, D.M. Medeiros, K. Lin and B.M. Thorne, Nutr.Res., 1984, 4, 305.
87. F.J. Kok, C.M. Van Duijn, A. Hofman, G.B. Van der Voet, F.A. De Wolff, C.H.C. Paays and H.A. Valkenburg, Am.J.Epidemiol., 1988, 128, 352.
88. N.W. Solomons, J.Am.Coll.Nutr., 1985, 4, 83.
89. D. Kromhout, A.A.E. Wibowo, R.F.M. Herber, L.M. Dalderup, H. Heerdink, C. de Coulander and R.L. Zielhuis, Am.J.Epidemiol., 1985, 122, 378.
90. S. Reiser, A. Powell, C. Yang and J.J. Canary, Nutr.Rep.Int., 1987, 36, 641.
91. D.M. Roden, Am.J.Cardiol., 1989, 63, 43G.
92. H. Ebel and T. Günther, J.Clin.Chem.Clin.Biochem., 1983, 21, 249.
93. H.S. Rasmussen, P. Aurup, S. Hojberg, E.K. Jensen and P. McNair, Arch.Intern.Med., 1986, 146, 872.
94. J. Sheehan, Am.J.Cardiol., 1989, 63, 35G.
95. H.S. Rasmussen, P. McNair, P. Norregard, V. Backer, O. Lindeneg and S. Balslev, Lancet, 1986, i, 234.
96. A.S. Abraham, D. Rosenmann, M. Kramer, J. Balkin, M.M. Zion, H. Farbstien and U. Eylath, Arch.Intern.Med., 1987, 147, 753.
97. B.C. Morton, R.C. Nair, F.M. Smith, T.G. McKibbon and W.J. Poznanski, Magnesium, 1984, 3, 346.
98. L.F. Smith, A.M. Heagerty, R.F. Bing and D.B. Barnett, Int.J.Cardiol., 1986, 12, 175.
99. B.M. Altura, Magnesium, 1988, 7, 57.
100. A. Sjögren, L. Edvinsson and B. Fallgren, J.Intern.Med., 1989, 226, 213.

101. H. Luoma, S.K.J. Helminen, H. Ranta, I. Rytömaa and J.H. Meurman, Scand.J.Clin.Lab.Invest., 1973, 32, 217.
102. D.R. Taves, Nature, 1978, 272, 361.
103. M.L. Bierenbaum, A.I. Fleischman, R. Stein and T. Hayton, J.Med.Soc.N.J., 1974, 71, 663.
104. G.K. Tokuhata, E. Digon and K. Ramaswamy, Public Health Rep., 1978, 93, 60.
105. S.L. Miller, J.Public Health Dent., 1980, 40, 346.
106. J.M. Nixon and R.G. Carpenter, Lancet, 1974, ii, 1068.
107. H. Luoma, A. Aromaa, S. Helminen, H. Murtomaa, L. Kiviluoto, S. Punsar and P. Knekt, Acta Med.Scand., 1983, 213, 171.
108. Steering Committee of the Physicians' Health Study Research Group, N.Engl.J.Med., 1989, 321, 129.
109. P.M. Farrell, "Vitamin E: A Comprehensive Treatise", L.J. Machlin, ed., Marcel Dekker, Inc., New York, 1980, p. 520.
110. K. Haeger, Vasa, 1973, 2, 280.
111. A. Vogelsang and E.V. Shute, Nature, 1946, 157, 772.
112. K.F. Gey, H.P. Stähelin, P. Puska and A. Evans, Ann.N.Y.Acad.Sci., 1987, 498, 110.
113. K.F. Gey, P. Puska, P. Jordan and U.K. Moser, Am.J.Clin.Nutr., 1990, in press.
114. M. Okuma, H. Takayama and H. Uchino, Prostaglandins, 1980, 19, 527.
115. J.S.C. Fong, Experientia, 1976, 32, 639.
116. J.A.C. Gomes, D. Venkatachalapathy and J.I. Haft, Am.Heart.J., 1976, 91, 425.
117. M.J. Stampfer, J.A. Jakubowski, D. Faigel, R. Vaillancourt and D. Deykin, Am.J.Clin.Nutr., 1988, 47, 700.
118. C. Colette, N. Pares-Herbute, L.H. Monnier and E. Cartry, Am.J.Clin.Nutr., 1988, 47, 256.
119. S. Renaud, M. Ciavatti, L. Perrot, F. Berthezene, D. Dargent and P. Condamin, Contraception, 1987, 36, 347.
120. A. Bendich and L.J. Machlin, Am.J.Clin.Nutr., 1988, 48, 612.
121. W.J.Hermann, Jr., K. Ward and J. Faucett, Am.J.Clin.Pathol., 1979, 72, 848.
122. D. Steinberg, S. Parthasarathy, T.E. Carew, J.C. Khoo and J.L. Witztum, N.Engl.J.Med., 1989, 320, 915.
123. W. Jessup, S.M. Rankin, C.V. De Whalley, J.R.S. Hoult, J. Scott and D.S. Leake, Biochem.J., 1990, 265, 399.
124. D.W. Morel, J.R. Hessler and G.M. Chisolm, J.Lipid Res., 1983, 24, 1070.
125. D.W. Morel and G.M. Chisolm, J. Lipid Res., 1989, 30, 1827.
126. E. Ginter, Adv. Lipid Res., 1978, 16, 167.
127. G.E. Johnson and S.S. Obenshain, Am.J.Clin.Nutr., 1981, 34, 2088.

128. G. Wahlberg and G. Walldius, Atherosclerosis, 1982, 43, 283.
129. N. Bishop, C.J. Schorah and J.K. Wales, Diabetic Med., 1985, 2, 121.
130. A. Aro, M. Kyllästinen, E. Kostiainen, C.G. Gref, S. Elfving and U. Uusitalo, Ann.Nutr.Metab., 1988, 32, 133.

The Epidemiology of Selenium and Human Cancer

W. C. Willett, M. J. Stampfer, D. Hunter, and G. A. Colditz

FROM THE DEPARTMENTS OF EPIDEMIOLOGY AND NUTRITION, HARVARD SCHOOL OF PUBLIC HEALTH, AND THE CHANNING LABORATORY, DEPARTMENT OF MEDICINE, HARVARD MEDICAL SCHOOL AND BRIGHAM AND WOMEN'S HOSPITAL, BOSTON, MA, USA

1 INTRODUCTION

A substantial body of evidence indicates that selenium supplementation can decrease cancer incidence in a variety of laboratory animals.[1] However, in a few animal models, selenium supplements have increased tumour incidence.[2] In several of the studies, interactions of selenium with other nutrients have been observed, including vitamin A[3] and vitamin E[4] which produced synergistic effects, and vitamin C,[5] which manifested an antagonistic effect. The plausibility that higher selenium intake might reduce cancer incidence has been greatly enhanced by elucidation of its function as a component of glutathione peroxidase, an enzyme with an important antioxidant role.[6]

These animal experiments have spurred a number of studies in humans. We will here review evidence that bears on an association between selenium and human cancer, using data from geographical, case-control, and prospective studies.

2 GEOGRAPHICAL STUDIES

More than 20 years ago, Shamberger and Frost suggested[7] that total cancer mortality rates in the United States were inversely correlated with selenium exposure, as reflected by levels in plants.[8] In subsequent work, Shamberger et al. calculated age-specific rates for white males 55-64 years of age by states categorized according to one of four levels of selenium concentration in forage crops; a monotonic trend of increasing cancer rates with lower levels of selenium was observed. These authors also examined the association between selenium concentrations in donated blood samples from 19 cities in the United States and age-specific cancer death rates, observing a correlation of -0.49, $p<0.05$.[9] These findings were replicated by Clark et al. cited secondarily[10] who

---

Supported in part by research grants (CA42182 and CA42059) from the National Institutes of Health

based the analyses on county rather than state, controlled for urbanization and several other potential confounders, and used a method to give greater weight to counties with larger populations and more stable death rates. Similar inverse relationships were seen in a reanalysis using more recent U.S. cancer mortality data[11], and within the state of Texas for all sites,[12] and within New York State for colorectal cancer[13].

Schrauzer et al. noted remarkably high inverse correlations between calculated per capita dietary selenium consumption and cancer mortality rates in different countries, particularly for breast ($r=-0.80$) and colon ($r=-0.73$). Similar findings were observed using mean selenium levels in donor blood; correlations were $r=-0.76$ for breast and $r=-0.68$ for colon cancer. The correlations between mean donor blood selenium concentration and cancer mortality within the United States were similar to the international data: for breast cancer $r=-0.70$, and for colon cancer $r=-0.69$.[14]

In a Chinese study, the mean blood selenium concentrations in samples drawn from healthy adults in 24 regions were examined in relation to the corresponding cancer mortality rates. Strong inverse correlations were observed for overall cancer mortality ($r=-0.62$), particularly for stomach and esophagus.[15] Guo et al.[16] have recently analysed data on pooled plasma selenium levels from 65 counties in China in relation to esophageal cancer mortality rates. Correlations were -0.22 for males and -0.26 for females ($p<0.10$ for both); somewhat stronger inverse correlations were seen for vitamin C and fruit intake but multivariate analyses were not provided adjusting the association with selenium levels for these other variables. Notably, cancer of the stomach and esophagus were not significantly correlated with selenium in the study by Schrauzer et al.[13] However, in a study from South Africa, whole blood selenium levels were lower among Blacks in rural areas with high rates of esophageal cancer than in rural and urban areas with low rates of this cancer.[17]

These geographical studies have been an important stimulus for research. However, other factors, such as diet, which differ among these regions could account for the association with selenium. Countries with high estimated selenium intake are typically the less affluent countries which differ in many respects from economically advanced countries. The inverse associations within countries provides greater support for the hypothesis. Case-control and cohort studies afford greater control of potential confounding variables.

3 CASE-CONTROL STUDIES

In case-control studies, cancer patients and healthy individuals are compared with respect to their selenium status. Because selenium in foods varies considerably depending upon the levels in the soil, a calculated dietary assessment would, under most conditions, provide a poor measurement of individual selenium intake. Thus, nearly all published studies to date have used blood (or tissue) levels as a measure of selenium status. In most of these case-control studies selenium levels have been lower among cancer patients,[17-28] although there were some inconsistent results for specific cancer sites. For example, Shamberger et al. found a significantly reduced selenium level in six cases of Hodgkin's disease, but not among other lymphoproliferative disorders,[17] whereas Calautti found normal levels in 20 Hodgkin's disease patients, and decreased levels in four patients with chronic lymphocytic leukemia.[22] Similarly, for breast cancer, Shamberger et al. found no difference (11 cases),[17] but McConnell et al. observed lower levels in 35 cases than in 27 controls.[21] Schrauzer et al. measured blood selenium levels in breast cancer cases and controls in the United States and Japan, and found significantly lower levels in the cases in both countries,[26] but, few details were provided on selection procedures and the stage of disease among the cases. Basu et al.[28] reported a nonsignificant mean lower serum selenium level among 30 women with breast cancer than among 30 controls. In most studies that examined gastrointestinal cancer, lower levels were found among cases[17,19,21,27] but not in all instances.[24]

In several case-control studies, no overall decrease in selenium levels was found among cancer cases.[29-32] Broghamer et al. observed increased levels of serum selenium among 59 patients with reticuloendothelial cancer (including Hodgkin's disease) which was interpreted as a treatment effect.[29] In a case-control study in New Zealand, where levels of selenium are very low, 80 cancer patients were observed to have levels similar to controls.[30] In two other small studies in women (23 cases total), no material differences were found between cancer cases and controls.[31,32] In a study by Meyer and Verreault,[33] 38 early stage breast cancer cases and controls had similar serum selenium levels. In a preliminary report of a Dutch study of 134 cases of breast cancer and 289 control women, no differences were observed for selenium measured in plasma, erythrocytes, or toenails.[34] Goodwin et al. found that cases of oral cancer had lower levels of erythrocyte selenium than controls, but higher plasma selenium levels.[35] In preliminary findings from a case-control study in South Dakota, an area with unusually high but variable soil selenium levels, no reduction in risk of breast (138 cases) and colon or rectum cancer (126 cases) was observed among persons with high toenail levels.[36] For lung cancer, a significant inverse association was seen for men (77 cases), but not for women (35 cases).

The findings of the case-control studies are suggestive of a possible protective affect of selenium for several cancer sites, but difficult to interpret. Most of the investigations included only a small number of subjects; only two had more than 100 cases. In many instances, little attention was given to possible confounding. However, the major limitation inherent in the case-control design is the possibility that the disease or its treatment can influence selenium levels measured after diagnosis. Selenium can be concentrated in certain tumours, depriving the host tissues and perhaps thereby reducing circulating levels; this has been observed in animal[37] and human tumours.[38] However, it is unlikely that this property alone could account for lower serum levels except perhaps for a massive tumour. More likely to be important is the effect of cancer (and its treatment) on general nutritional status. Cancer often leads to a decline in intake of many nutrients, and their blood levels are often reduced. Two studies which examined the selenium status of cancer patients longitudinally found that blood levels declined as the disease progressed.[30,39] Three case-control studies with positive results found that patients with more advanced disease had lower selenium levels.[17,19,40]

The influence of the cancer on selenium status in a case-control study can be minimized by selecting cases with small tumours at sites unlikely to have systemic effects. Clark et al.[41] used this approach in studying patients with basal and squamous cell skin cancer. They found a strong and highly significant inverse relation between plasma selenium and skin cancer. Relative risks ranged from three to six for extreme deciles, depending upon the histological type and the control group chosen for analysis. Similarly, Dawson et al.[42] reported preliminary results of a study of 36 women with cervical hyperplasia; these women had significantly lower levels of serum selenium than controls. Also, using a premalignant lesion as an endpoint, Dworkin et al.[40] found that 37 patients with adenomatous colon polyps had plasma and erythrocyte selenium levels similar to those of control patients. In a German case-control study[43] 101 melanoma patients had a mean serum selenium level (69.6 $\pm$ 1.2) significantly lower than that of 80 control subjects (81.2 $\pm$ 2.0). The appropriateness of the control subjects, however, is unclear as they were said to be randomly selected healthy volunteers, without specification of the sampling frame. Although state III cancers had the lowest levels, case - control differences also existed for cancers with localized disease. A different approach to reduce potential impact of malignancy on selenium measurement was used by Jaskiewicz et al.[17] in a case-control study of esophageal cancer in South Africa. Instead of measuring levels in the cases themselves, whole blood selenium levels of household members of 19 cases were compared with age-sex matched persons in 49 households without esophageal cancer; significantly lower values were found for the case households.

Another approach for minimizing the influence of disease on selenium measurements in case-control studies is to analyse levels in a tissue that reflects intake well before the cancer diagnosis. We have previously demonstrated that selenium concentrates in the nails, and that the levels reflect dietary intake.[44,45] Clippings from a single toenail represent tissue levels at the time the nail was formed, integrated over several weeks. Because of the variable length of nails, clippings from all ten toes represent tissue levels from a time-integrated period of approximately five to twelve months prior to clipping; clippings from the great toe alone may be particularly useful in the context of a case-control study. For this reason, nail clippings were used in our case-control study in South Dakota and in the Dutch study by van't Veer et al.[34]

4 PROSPECTIVE STUDIES

The most direct way to minimize the possibility that cancer may alter the selenium level is by conducting prospective studies in which the tissue samples are collected before the onset of disease. The major disadvantage of this approach is that even over a number of years, the risk for any individual of developing cancer is quite low. Hence, samples must be collected from many subjects who are then followed for years to identify diagnoses of cancer. Prospective investigations can be efficient if they utilize samples that have been already collected and stored for other purposes. By analysing the levels of individuals who subsequently developed cancer, and a sample of those who remained healthy, one obtains nearly all the information as a study analysing every sample at the outset, but at far lower cost. All but one of the reported prospective studies of selenium and cancer have employed this design, sometimes called a case-control study nested in a cohort.

In the first prospective study of selenium and cancer,[46] Willett et al. analysed sera which had been collected in 1973 as part of the Hypertension Detection and Follow-up Program (HDFP), a trial of hypertension treatment. Samples were available from 4480 subjects from 14 centers across the United States, of whom 111 developed cancer (excluding nonmelanoma skin cancer) in the ensuing five years. Two controls were matched to each case by age, sex, smoking history, month of blood collection, initial blood pressure, use of antihypertensive medication, randomization assignment, and (in women) menopausal status and parity. Sera were assayed by neutron activation analysis.[47] There was a small but statistically significant difference in mean selenium level between individuals who subsequently developed cancer (129 ± SEM 2 µg/L) and those who remained free of cancer (136 ± 2, p=0.02). The excess risk was most pronounced among those in the lowest quintile of serum selenium, for whom the relative risk, compared to the highest three quintiles (based on the control distribution) was 1.9 (95% confidence limits (CL) 1.1, 3.3). The mean values were lower for all specific cancer sites, as compared with controls; the strongest association appeared to be for a heterogeneous group of gastrointestinal cancers (13 cases). The weakest association was for breast cancer (16 cases).

Four subsequent prospective studies employing a similar design have been reported from Finland; two by Salonen and colleagues,[48,49] and others by Virtamo et al.[50] and Knekt et al.[51,52] These are of particular interest because Finland is a known low selenium area. The first study[48] included 128 cancer cases, 59 men and 69 women, matched to controls (1:1) by age, sex, tobacco use, and serum cholesterol level. The mean serum selenium level for those who subsequently developed cancer was 50.5 ± 1.1 µg/L, as compared with 54.3 ± 1.0 for those who remained healthy (p=0.01). The excess risk was concentrated among those with the lower selenium levels. Individuals in the bottom 30% of the distribution (cases and controls combined) had a relative risk of 3.1 (95% CL 1.5, 6.7) compared to those in the upper 70%. The differences were most pronounced for gastrointestinal, respiratory, and hematological malignancies, as well as cancers of miscellaneous sites. No material differences were observed for urogenital, skin, skeletal, or breast cancers.

The second Finnish study[49] was conducted in the same region of Finland, using a similar study design in a different cohort. The mean selenium level among 51 individuals who subsequently developed, and died of, cancer was 53.7 ± 1.8 µg/L, as compared to 60.9 ± 1.8 for matched controls who remained cancer free, p=0.02. The relative risk of those in the lower third of the distribution (case and control combined) was 5.8 (95% CL 1.2, 2.9) as compared to the others with higher values.

The third Finnish study, by Virtamo et al.[50], was conducted among 1110 men in two rural areas of Finland who were followed for nine years. Mean serum selenium values were 53.9 µg/L for those with 109 incident cancers and 55.3 for those remaining without cancer, these values were not significantly different. A significantly lower mean value (49.4 µg/L) was seen among the 37 men with prevalent cancer at baseline or who were diagnosed within one year of blood collection, consistent with an effect of cancer on selenium status.

A more recent Finnish study[51] evaluated serum selenium levels in relation to 150 incident gastrointestinal cancers developing among 36,265 men and women during 6-10 years of follow-up. Serum selenium values were 11.7% higher among controls than cases of esophageal or gastric cancer in men (mean, 58.9 µg/L for cases) and 6.8% higher in women (mean for cases, 60.7 µg/L). For lowest compared with highest tertiles, the relative risk was 2.2 for men (p trend = 0.001) and 1.5 for women without a significant trend. These relative risks were not reduced by eliminating cases diagnosed within two years of follow-up. Among women, controlling simultaneously for smoking, serum cholesterol, alpha-tocopherol, and ß-carotene reduced the relative risk to 1.0. No associations were observed between selenium levels and incidence of colorectal cancer (21 cases in men and 36 in women). Another recent report using the same collection of sera included data for other cancer sites.[52] For all cancers combined, the differences for men between mean levels among cases (60.7 µg/L $\pm$ 19.0) compared with controls (64.4 $\pm$ 17.7) was statistically significant, whereas the mean values for women (61.9 $\pm$ 14.0 for cases vs 63.0 $\pm$ 15.2) were not significantly different. Among men, smoking-adjusted relative risks for the highest four quintiles compared with the lowest quintile were strongest for pancreas (RR = 0.25, p>0.05; 189 cases), and basal cell skin cancer (RR = 0.58, p>0.05, 64 cases). Little association was seen for cancer of the prostate (51 cases), urinary tract (34 cases) or breast cancer in women (90 cases). Exclusion of the first two years of follow-up did not appreciably alter the findings.

In an extension of the nonmelanoma skin cancer case-control study cited earlier[41], Clark et al.[53] prospectively studied 177 patients among whom 19 developed recurrent nonmelanoma skin cancer. The relative risk for levels above versus below the median was 0.8.

Evans County, Georgia, one of the HDFP centers, was the site of a separate prospective study.[54] Blood samples were drawn in 1967-69 from 2530 individuals, of whom 130 subsequently developed cancer. Each case was matched to two controls by race, age, sex, and time of venipuncture. The mean selenium levels among those who developed cancer was 116 µg/L, and for those who remained healthy was 115. The extreme quartiles had no difference in risk and no material associations were seen for any specific cancer sites.

Menkes et al.[55] conducted a similar analysis for lung cancer alone, using blood drawn from 25,802 residents of Washington County, Maryland in 1974. During eight years of follow-up, 99 individuals developed lung cancer and were matched 1:2 to controls by age, sex, race, smoking history, and month of blood collection. Cases had nonsignificantly higher mean serum selenium levels (113 µg/L) than did controls (110 µg/L). In contrast to other studies, there was a trend for increasing risk with higher quintile level of selenium (p=0.07). The relative risk for the upper half as compared to the lower half of the selenium levels was 4.2 (95% CL 1.4, 12.5) for squamous cell, 1.3 (0.5, 3.6) for small cell, 1.4 (0.6, 3.3) for adenocarcinoma, and 3.7 (1.0, 14.3) for large cell and unspecified type.

In another analysis based on sera from Washington County, Helzlsouer et al.[56] observed lower selenium levels for 35 incident cases of bladder cancer (mean = 111 + 11) compared with those of 70 matched controls (mean = 117 + 13 p=0.03). The relative risk for the lowest compared with the highest tertile of selenium level was 2.06. An inverse association was also noted for 22 cases of pancreatic cancer occurring in this cohort.[57] Mean levels were 125 for cases and 141 for matched controls (p=0.025); a significant apparent protective effect persisted after controlling for other nutritional variables and smoking. The relation between serum selenium level and risk of colon cancer in this cohort was examined by Schober et al.[58] The mean level for 72 cases was 110 and for 143 matched controls was 115 (p=0.07). The relative risk for those in the highest compared with the lowest quintile was 0.7 (95% confidence interval = 0.3-1.7). Even though this analysis included more colon cancer cases than most other cohorts, the imprecision can be appreciated by noting that, despite not being statistically significant, the study is statistically compatible with a greater than 70% reduction in risk among those in the highest quintile compared with the lowest.

Kok et al.[59] analysed sera from a cohort of 10,532 men and women, of whom 69 died of cancer after the first year of follow-up. Cases were matched 1:2 to controls by age, sex, and smoking. Among the 40 men, the mean level for cases (117 µg/L) was significantly lower than controls (126), p=0.04, and the relative risk for the lowest quintile, compared to higher levels, was 2.7 (95% CI 1.2, 6.2). Female cases, however, had slightly higher levels (131) than controls (129) and a relative risk for the lowest quintile of 1.5 (0.5, 4.5). For the total group, the relative risk was 1.9 (1.0, 3.5).

Blood was drawn from 6860 men in the Honolulu Heart Program who were followed for nine years; 280 cases of cancer were diagnosed during this period. Among those who subsequently became cases, the mean serum selenium level was 123 ± 20 (standard deviation) and among a random sample of controls of comparable age the mean was 125 ± 19.[60] No material differences were observed for any specific cancer site: bladder (n=29), rectum (n=32), colon (n=82), stomach (n=66), or lung (n=71). For lung cancer, there was a slight trend towards protection with lower levels of selenium, as seen by Menkes et al.[55], but this did not approach significance, p=0.41; the relative risk for the lowest tertile was 0.8 compared with the highest.

In preliminary results from the Multiple Risk Factor Intervention Trial (MRFIT), no association was seen between selenium level and subsequent occurrence of cancer.[61] The 156 cases of cancer (including 70 lung cancers) were matched by age, clinic, and smoking status to controls; there were no material associations with serum selenium for all cancer sites combined or for lung cancer alone.

Coates et al.[62], using sera collected and stored from 6,167 men and women living in Washington State, identified 154 incident cancers and compared prediagnostic selenium levels (mean = 162 µg/L) with those of 282 controls (mean = 162). (For a few subjects and their matched controls, plasma rather than serum was available.) Relative risks comparing highest with lowest tertiles of blood selenium levels were 1.0 for gastrointestinal cancers (28 cases), 3.4 for breast (20 cases), 0.3 for prostate (13 cases), 0.6 of lymphoma or leukemia (12 cases), 1.1 cervix (12 cases), 0.8 for lung (11 cases) and 0.9 for other cancer (58 cases).

In a study from northern Norway, Ringstad et al.[63] identified 60 incident cases of cancer during six years of follow-up among 9,364 men and women who were 20-54 years of age at the time of blood collection. The mean serum selenium levels in cases (123.2 µg/L) was similar to that of controls (128.7). However, for the 25 fatal cancers, selenium levels in serum collected before diagnosis was significantly lower than for their matched controls.

Van Noord et al.[64] collected toenail clippings from 8,760 premenopausal women in Holland and identified 34 prevalent breast cancer cases and 27 subsequent cases during up to four years of follow-up. Mean selenium levels for these cases were similar to those of matched controls; the relative risk for highest vs lowest quintiles was 1.1 (95% CI 0.5-2.9) for both case groups combined.

Hunter et al.[65] reported preliminary analyses using toenail specimens collected from 68,213 U.S. women in the Nurses' Health Study during 1982-83. During four years of follow-up 393 women were diagnosed with breast cancer and were matched to 393 control women by age and month of nail collection. Median values for cases (0.787 ppm) and for controls (0.788) were virtually identical. The relative risk for the highest compared with lowest quintile was 1.11 (95% CI=0.72-1.72). The large number of cases makes an important relation between selenium intake and breast cancer unlikely. An important element of this study was a repeated collection of nail samples among a subset of women 6 years after the original collection. The positive correlation (r=0.60) over this period indicates that a single nail specimen does provide an index of intake over many years.

In all these prospective studies, blood or nail samples were collected prior to the diagnosis of disease. However, the possibility remains that the levels may have been influenced by preclinical disease, which would tend to yield a spurious inverse association between selenium level and risk of cancer. Most studies addressed this possibility by examining the levels among cases at various time intervals since the blood was drawn; in none of the studies with positive findings was there any indication that such a spurious effect was present.

The prospective studies of selenium and cancer have yielded conflicting results. One possible explanation for the inconsistent results is that perhaps studies with the null findings did not include an adequate range of values to observe a difference. Because a potentially important source of variation in selenium levels is due to geographically-determined soil levels, this problem may be more severe in studies limited to one city as opposed to a national sample. There is some support for this suggestion.

In general among studies using sera, those with positive results had coefficients of variation of 20.4% or more, whereas those with null or negative results had values of 17.4% or less.[66] One might expect that the MRFIT study would have a reasonably wide range of levels since participants were drawn from clinics at various locations in the US. However, in these analyses the controls were matched to cases within clinic, constraining them towards similar values. Indeed, this consideration provided the rationale in the HDFP study to specifically avoid matching by clinic. In addition, any relation between selenium intake and cancer incidence is likely to be non-linear with greatest risk among the lowest extreme of intake. The greater consistency of inverse associations in studies from Finland, where intake has been quite low, is compatible with the notion that only very low intake increases risk of cancer. Kok et al.[59] have raised the possibility that selenium may be protective only in men, not in women. Of the studies with overall positive results, those that examined the data separately by gender[46,48,51,59] failed to find a significant or material effect among women.

The limited numbers of cancers at any specific site within nearly all studies is likely to contribute to apparent inconsistency because there is no reason to believe that selenium would have a similar association with all types of cancer. The number of cancers needed to be confident that no important association exists can be appreciated if we assume that a 30% reduction in risk for the highest compared with lowest quintile would be of interest (this difference in levels could be achieved by supplementation). Only the Nurses' Health Study, with approximately 400 cases of breast cancer, had sufficient precision so that the lower bound 95% confidence interval of a null association excluded a 30% reduction in risk. These data as well as several other null studies with a substantial number of breast cancer cases[34,36,52] conducted in low[52] as well as high[36] selenium areas, provide reasonable confidence that a beneficial effect for breast cancer large enough to justify considering supplementation does not exist. There is no other site with sufficient data to make a similar null statement. The sites for which selenium appears most promising as a beneficial agent are probably cancer of the stomach and esophagus, pancreas, and possibly lung (although several null studies have been published). Minimal data are available for prostate cancer.

If selenium status is indeed associated with risk of cancer, the dose-response considerations present a puzzling phenomenon in that virtually the entire Finnish population (and that of New Zealand as well) falls into the lowest quintile of the US population, as defined in the HDFP data. Although cancer rates, especially of the breast and colon, are high in all three countries, they are not dramatically different. One possible explanation is that the HDFP results represent a chance finding, and selenium levels that prevail in the US are actually not related to cancer risk. Another possibility that we have discussed in detail elsewhere[66] is that serum selenium represents a two compartment system, such that levels of the active compartment may overlap considerably between the US and Finland, whereas the larger, passive component (reflected in the overall serum level) has little overlap.

The potential for interaction between nutrients presents a further degree of complexity in interpreting the data on selenium and cancer. As mentioned earlier, there are ample data from animal studies demonstrating interactions between selenium and vitamin A[2] and vitamin E.[3] Several of the prospective studies have investigated possible nutrient interactions. In the HDFP study, the strongest effect of selenium appeared among those with the lowest levels of serum retinol or vitamin E or both.[46]

Similar findings were observed by Kok et al.[59] A strong interaction with vitamin E, though not with vitamin A, was reported from the second Finnish Study.[49] Although interactions were not statistically significant Knekt[52] found that selenium was most strongly associated with lower cancer risk among persons with lower serum alpha-tocopherol or ß-carotene levels. In contrast, Menkes et al.[55] found that the combination of low vitamin E and high serum selenium led to increased risk of lung cancer. Clark et al.[53] found that the protective association with selenium was present only among those with low levels of total carotenoids; vitamin E was not assayed. The Hawaii study, in which both vitamins A and E were measured, failed to observe such an interaction.

5 SUMMARY

The rapid accumulation of data over the last few years has provided increasing refinement of our knowledge regarding the relation of selenium levels and cancer risk. We can be reasonably certain that higher levels do not uniformly reduce the risk of all cancer sites. For one important site, breast cancer, we can be quite confident that an important association does not exist, except perhaps with extremely high intakes or with a very long latent period. This finding is notable, as geographic correlations have been particularly strong for this malignancy. No firm conclusion can be reached for other sites; an adequate resolution will probably require studies that include hundreds of cases for a specific cancer site. The most promising associations have been seen for cancers of the esophagus and stomach. Protective association have also been seen for lung cancer in several studies, although no association has been observed in other investigations. For these specific sites the potential for confounding by cigarette smoking, alcohol intake, and other dietary factors is particularly great and must be seriously considered in the design of studies. If any randomized trial is to be considered, it should be conducted among men with relatively low tissue selenium levels and at high risk of these particular malignancies.

6 REFERENCES

1. C. Ip, J. Am. Coll. Tox., 1986, 5, 7.
2. D.F. Birt, A.D. Julius, C.E. Runice, L.T. White, T. Lawson and P.M. Pour, Nutr. Cancer., 1988, 11, 21.
3. H.J. Thompson, L.D. Meeker, P. Becci, Can. Res., 1981, 41, 1413.
4. P.M. Horvath and C. Ip, Can. Res., 1983, 43, 5335.
5. M.M. Jacobs, Prev. Med., 1980, 9, 362.

6. W.G. Hoekstra, In 'Traced element metabolism in animals', W.G. Hoekstra, J.W. Suttre, H.G. Ganther and W. Mentz, eds., University Park Press, Baltimore, 1974, Vol. 2, p. 61.
7. R.J. Shamberger and D.V. Frost, Can. Med. Assoc. J., 1969, 100.
8. J. Kubota, W.H. Allaway, D.L. Carter, E.E. Cary and V.A. Lazar, J. Agric. Food. Chem., 1967, 15, 448.
9. R.J. Shamberger, S.A. Tytko and C.E. Willis, Arch. Env. Health, 1976, 31, 231.
10. L.C. Clark, Fed. Proc., 1985, 44, 2584.
11. U.M. Cowgill, Fed. Proc., 1985, 44, 2584.
12. I. Chech, A. Holguin, H. Sokolow and V. Smith, South Med. J., 1984, 77, 1415.
13. B. Jansson, Can. Prev. Detect., 1985, 8, 341.
14. G.N. Schrauzer, D.A. White and C.J. Schneider, Bioinorg. Chem., 1977, 7, 23.
15. S. Yu, Y. Chu, X. Gong and C. Hou, Bio. Trace Element Res., 1985, 7, 21.
16. W. Guo, J.Y. Li, W.J. Blot, A.W. Hsing, J. Chen and J.F. Fraumeni Jr., Nutr. Cancer, 1990, 13, 121.
17. K. Jaskiewicz, W.F.O. Marasas, J.E. Rossouw, F.E. Van Niekerk and E.P.W. Heine Tech, Cancer, 1988, 62, 2635.
18. R.J. Shamberger, E. Rukovena, A.K. Longfield, S.A. Tytko, S. Deodhar and C.E. Willis, J. Natl. Cancer Inst., 1973, 50, 863.
19. K.P. McConnell, W.L. Broghamer, A.L. Blotcky and O.J. Hurt, J. Nutr., 1975, 105, 1026.
20. W.L. Broghamer, K.P. McConnell and A.L. Blotcky, Cancer, 1976, 37, 1384.
21. K.P. McConnell, R.M. Jager, K.I. Bland and A.J. Blotcky, J. Surg. Oncol., 1980, 15, 67.
21. P. Calautti, G. Moschini, B.M. Stievano, L. Tomio, F. Calzavara and G. Perona, Scand. J. Haematol., 1980, 24, 63.
23. Y. Hojo, Bull. Environ. Contam. Toxicol., 1981, 26, 466.
24. L. Gerhardsson, D. Brune, I.G.F. Nordberg and P.O. Wester, Br. J. Ind. Med., 1985, 42, 617.
25. H. Sundstrom, O. Ylikorkala and A. Kauppila, Carcinogenesis, 1986, 7, 1051.
26. G.N. Schrauzer, T. Molenaar, S. Mead, K. Kuehn, H. Yamamoto and E. Araki, Jpn. J. Can. Res., 1985, 76, 374.
27. L. Pothier, W.L. Lane, A. Bhargava, C. Michielson and H.O. Douglass Jr., Cancer, 1987, 60, 2251.
28. T.K. Basu, G.B. Hill, D. Ng, E. Abdi and N. Temple, J. Am. Coll. Nutr., 1989, 8, 524.
29. W.L. Broghamer, K.P. McConnell, M. Grimaldi and A.J. Blotcky, Cancer, 1978, 41, 1462.
30. M.F. Robinson, P.J. Godfrey, C.D. Thomson, H.M. Rea and A.M. van Rij, Am. J. Clin. Nutr., 1979, 32, 1477.
31. T.D. Schultz and J.E. Leklem, Am. J. Clin. Nutr., 1983, 37, 114.

32. L.N. Vernie, M. De Vries, C. Benckhuijsen, J.J.M. DeGoeij and C. Zegers, Cancer Lett., 1983, 18, 283.
33. F. Meyer and R. Verreault. Am. J. Epidemiol., 1987, 125, 917.
34. P. van't Veer, F.J. Kok, R.J.J. Hermus and F. Sturmans, Am. J. Epidemiol., 1989, 130, 811 (abstract).
35. W.J. Goodwin, W.H. Lane, K. Bradford, M.V. Marshall, A.C. Griffin, H. Geopfert and R.H. Jesse, Cancer, 1983, 51, 110.
36. C. Poole, 'Cancer and high selenium intake', Doctoral Thesis, Harvard School of Public Health, 1989.
37. W.A. Baumgartner, V.A. Hilla and E.T. Wright, Am. J. Clin. Nutr., 1978, 31, 457.
38. S.L. Rizk and H.H. Sky-Peck, Can. Res., 1984, 44, 5390.
39. H. Sundström, E. Yrjänheikki and A. Kauppila, Carcinogenesis, 1984, 44, 5390.
40. B.M. Dworkin, W.S. Rosenthal, A. Mittelman, L. Weiss, L. Applebee-Brady and Z. Arlin, Am. J. Gastroenterol., 1988, 83, 748.
41. L.C. Clark, G.F. Graham, K.G. Crounse, R. Grimson, B. Hulka and C.M. Shy, Nutr. Cancer, 1984, 6, 13.
42. E.B. Dawson, J.T. Nosovitch and E.V. Hannigan, Fed. Proc., 1984, 43, 612 (abstract).
43. U. Reinhold, H. Biltz, W. Bayer and K.H. Schmidt, Acta. Derm. Venereol., 1989, 69, 132.
44. J.S. Morris, M.J. Stampfer and W.C. Willett, Bio. Trace Element Res., 1983, 5, 529.
45. 1C.A. Swanson, M.P. Longnecker, C. Veillon, et al., Am. J. Clin. Nutr., in press.
46. W.C. Willett, B.F. Polk and J.S. Morris, Lancet, 1983, 2, 130.
47. D.M. McKown and J.S. Morris, J. Radioanal. Chem., 1978, 43, 411.
48. J.T. Salonen, G. Alfthan, J.K. Huttunen and P. Puska, Am. J. Epidemiol., 1984, 120, 342.
49. J.T. Salonen, R. Salonen, R. Lappalainen, P.H. Mäenpaa, G. Alfthan and P. Puska, Br. Med. J., 1985, 290, 417.
50. J. Virtamo, E Valkeila, G. Alfthan, S. Punsar, J.K. Huttunen and M.J. Karvonen, Cancer, 1987, 60, 145.
51. P. Knekt, A. Aromaa, J. Maatela, G. Alfthan, RK Aaran, L. Teppo and M. Hakama, Int. J. Cancer, 1988, 42, 846.
52. P. Knekt, A. Aromaa, J. Maatela, G. Alfthan, R.K. Aaran, M. Hakama, T. Hakulinen, R. Peto and L. Teppo, J. Nat. Can. Inst., 1990, 82, 864.
53. L.C. Clark, G. Graham and J. Bray, Am. J. Epidemiol., 1985, 122, 528 (abstract).
54. I. Peleg, S. Morris and C.G. Hames, Med. Oncol. Tumor Pharmacol., 1985, 2, 157.
55. M. Menkes, G. Comstock, J.P. Vuilleumier, K.J. Helsing, A.A. Rider and R. Brookmeyer, N. Engl. J. Med., 1986, 315, 1250.

56. K.J. Helzlsouer, G.W. Comstock and J.S. Morris, Can. Res., 1989, 49, 6144.
57. P.G.J. Burney, G.W. Comstock and J.S. Morris, Am. J. Clin. Nutr., 1989, 49, 895.
58. S.E. Schober, G.W. Comstock, K.J. Helsing, R.M. Salkeld, S.J. Morris, A.A. Rider and R. Brookmeyer, Am. J. Epidemiol., 1987, 126, 1033.
59. F.J. Kok, A.M. de Bruijn, A. Hofman, R. Vermeermen and H.A. Valkenburg. Am. J. Epidemiol., 1987, 125, 12.
60. A. Nomura, L.K. Heilbrun, J.S. Morris and N. Stemmermann, J. Nat. Can. Inst., 1988, in press.
61. L. Kuller. Pilot lung cancer trial. Presented at the Chemoprevention Clinical Trials Workshop, National Cancer Institute, May 11-12, 1987.
62. R.J. Coates, N.S. Weiss, J.R. Daling, J.S. Morris and R.F. Labbe. Am. J. Epidemiol., 1988, 128, 515.
63. J. Ringstad, B.K. Jacobsen, S. Tretli and Y. Thomassen, J. Clin. Pathol., 1988, 41, 454.
64. P.A.H. Van Noord, H.J.A. Collette, M.J. Maas and F. De Waard, Int. J. Epidemiol., 1987, 16, 318.
65. D.J. Hunter, J.S. Morris, M.J. Stampfer, G.A. Colditz, F.E. Speizer and W.C. Willett, Am. J. Epidemiol., 1989, 130, 810 (abstract).
66. W.C. Willett and M.J. Stampfer, Acta Pharmacol. et Toxicol., 1986, 59 (Suppl VII), 240.

Carcinogenicity and Teratogenicity of Metals

On the Carcinogenicity of Nickel and Chromium and their Compounds

A. Aitio[1] and L. Tomatis[2]

[1] INSTITUTE OF OCCUPATIONAL HEALTH, FINLAND
[2] INTERNATIONAL AGENCY FOR RESEARCH ON CANCER, FRANCE

1   INTRODUCTION

Several recent epidemiological and experimental studies have shed new light on the carcinogenic properties of nickel and its various compounds, and of chromium and its different compounds. Therefore, the International Agency for Research on Cancer in Lyons, France, performed new evaluations on the carcinogenicity to humans of these chemicals, and classified them accordingly[1], using criteria developed during the last 20 years. This paper reviews the pertinent findings, and the logic of these classifications.

2   NICKEL

Epidemiological Studies on Cancer

Nasal cancer among workers in nickel refineries was reported already in the 1930's[2], and conclusive evidence of an increased risk of lung and nasal sinus cancer was presented in 1958[3,4]. Several cohort studies have confirmed these findings thereafter. Practically nonexistent data on the nickel species present in the refinery dusts have, however, hampered the evaluation of the carcinogenic potency of different specific nickel compounds[5,6,7]. Recently, however, a re-evaluation of the exposures, together with a further follow-up of all the main cohorts in the different nickel refineries was undertaken[8], and this gave the opportunity to somewhat more specific evaluations[1], although it was realized that the estimations of exposure levels, and even of the species were rather crude, and not based on actual measurements, but on reconstructions based mainly on knowledge of the process chemistry.

Highest risks for lung and nasal cancers were observed among calcining workers, who were heavily

Table 1. Cancer risk (Standardized mortality ratio) for pulmonary and nasal sinus cancer in the four high-risk departments in the Clydach refinery among workers hired before 1930, with no less than 15 years' latency, and who worked less than one year in any other high risk department[8].

Work place	Estimated nickel exposure				Cancer SMR	
	Metallic	Sulfidic	Oxidic	Soluble	Lung	Sinus
Furnace	5.6	6.4	2.6	0.4	409	24800
Calcining	5.3	18.8	6.8	0.8	725	44500
Copper plant	–	13.1	0.4	1.1	317	13200
Hydrometallurgy	0.5	0.9	<0.1	1.3	196	18700

exposed to both nickel sulfides and oxides (Table 1). Exposures to oxides and sulfides coexisted in nickel refining, and therefore, it was not possible to differentiate the carcinogenic activities of the two. However, since there was a remarkably elevated risk for both lung and nasal cancer in the copper plant in the Clydach refinery (Table 1), where it was thought that the exposure to metallic nickel was negligible, it is evident that metallic nickel was not required for the carcinogenic effect.

High risks for both lung cancer and nasal sinus cancer were observed in the copper plant and hydrometallurgic department of the Clydach refinery, where the estimated exposures to oxidic (hydrometallurgy) and sulfidic nickel species (both hydrometallurgy and copper plant) were very much lower than those in the furnace and calcining areas, but exposures to soluble nickel species were high. The soluble nickel species handled in largest volumes here was nickel sulfate.

The notion of soluble nickel salts as causative factors behind lung and nasal sinus cancer was also corroborated by the findings in the Falconbridge refinery in Norway (Table 2), where highest risks of lung cancer were observed in the electrolytic department, and lower risks were observed in the calcining, roasting and smelting departments, where exposure was mainly to slightly soluble metallic, sulfidic and oxidic nickel species. Until the 1950's the main soluble salt in the electrolysis was nickel sulfate, thereafter it was nickel chloride, with some nickel sulfate.

No significant excess of respiratory tract cancer was observed in three studies of workers in high-nickel alloy manufacture or in a small study of users of metallic nickel powder; no increase in risk for lung cancer was observed in one small group of nickel elctroplaters not exposed to chromium.

Evaluation. The IARC working group concluded that there is **sufficient evidence** in humans for the carcinogenicity of nickel sulfate, and of the combinations of nickel sulfides and oxides encountered in the nickel refining industry, but that there is **inadequate evidence** for the carcinogenicity of metallic nickel and nickel alloys[1].

Table 2. Lung cancer risk (SMR) among workers in the Falconbridge nickel refinery, Norway, who had at least 5 years' work experience in the department, had not worked in the other high-risk department, and had no less than 15 years' latency period[8].

Work place	Estimated nickel exposure				Lung cancer
	Metallic	Sulfidic	Oxidic	Soluble	SMR
Calcining, roasting, smelting	<1.3	5-10	0.3	N	254
Electrolysis	<1.3	0.3-1.3	<1.3	1.3-5	476

Experimental studies on cancer[1].

Metallic nickel and nickel alloys. No study using inhalation exposure to **metallic nickel** demonstrated any carcinogenic activity. However, all these studies were limited because of poor survival of the animals; in a study with mice, all exposed animals died within 60 weeks, and in another with rats, 128/160 animals died by 15 months. Intratracheal instillation of metallic nickel produced adenocarcinomas and squamous cell carcinomas in a large proportion of the dosed rats, while none were seen in the controls. Subcutaneous, intramuscular and intrapleural administration of nickel powder or pellets induced sarcomas and carcinomas locally. In a preliminary study it was reported that a ferronickel alloy induced tumours after intratracheal administration in hamsters; different nickel alloys caused local sarcomas in three studies; in one study another alloy was not active.

Nickel oxides and hydroxides. Inhalation studies with nickel monoxide were not informative, because of small numbers of animals (rats), or because of poor survival (rats, hamsters). Ten intratracheal instillations of nickel monoxide induced a high frequency of pulmonary carcinomas in rats, intramuscular and intramuscular administrations induced local sarcomas in different strains of rats and mice; even intraperitoneal and intraperitoneal administration of nickel monoxide caused sarcomas in rats. In two limited studies in rats, nickel trioxide did not induce local tumours in rats. Crystalline nickel hydroxide, and nickel hydroxide gel induced local sarcomas in rats after intramuscular administration, whereas amorphous nickel hydroxide did not.

Nickel sulfides. Nickel subsulfide induced pulmonary adenomas and carcinomas after intratracheal administration in rats, and adeno- and squamous cell carcinomas after intratracheal instillation in rats. In induced local sarcomas after intrapleural, intramuscular, subcutaneous, intratesticular, intra-articular and retroperitoneal administration, as well as renal cell tumours after intrarenal, and various eye tumours of different origin after intraocular administration. After intramuscular implantation of millipore diffusion chambers containing nickel subsulfide, a high incidence of local sarcomas was induced. Nickel disulfide induced local tumours after intrarenal and intramuscular administration, and so did crystalline nickel monosulfide, while amorphous nickel monosulfide did not.

Nickel salts. Repeated intraperitoneal injections of nickel sulfate, nickel chloride and nickel acetate induced malignant tumours of the peritoneal cavity in rats; nickel acetate also induced lung adenocarcinomas in strain A mice.

Other nickel compounds. Nickel sulfarsenide, two nickel arsenides, nickel antimonide, nickel telluride and two different nickel selenides induced local sarcomas in rats after intramuscular administration, but not local tumours after intrarenal administration. Nickel monoarsenide and nickel titanate did not cause sarcomas after local administration.

Evaluation. The IARC working group concluded that there is **sufficient evidence** in experimental animals for the carcinogenicity of metallic nickel, nickel monoxides, nickel hydroxides and crystalline nickel sulfides, **limited evidence** for the carcinogenicity of nickel alloys, nickelocene, nickel carbonyl, nickel salts, nickel arsenides, nickel antimonide, nickel selenides and nickel telluride. The evidence was considered **inadequate** for the carcinogenicity of nickel trioxide, amorphous nickel sulfide and nickel titanate.

Other relevant data.

Nickel and its compounds were generally negative in tests for genotoxicity performed *in vivo*. However, *in vitro*, metallic nickel transformed animal cells, nickel oxides transformed cultured rodent cells, and induced anchorage-independent growth of human cells, and crystalline nickel subsulfide and sulfide were active in a variety of different tests with mammalian cells, and also induced gene mutation on *Paramoecium*. Nickel sulfate has been extensively studied for genotoxicity and related end-points in mammalian cells *in vitro*; it induced chromosomal aberrations and sister chromatid exchanges, transformed cultured cells, and produced gene mutation and DNA damage. Nickel sulfate also inhibited intercellular communication. Nickel chloride and acetate have been less extensively studied, but likewise, have been positive in all studies performed.

Overall evaluation

The IARC working group made the overall evaluation on nickel compounds as a group on the basis of the combined results of epidemiological studies – demonstrating conclusively the carcinogenicity of nickel sulfate and a combination of less soluble nickel sulfides and oxides – animal studies – demonstrating the carcinogenicity of several nickel compounds – and several types of other relevant data supported by the underlying concept that nickel compounds can generate nickel ions at critical sites in their target cells. The working group thus concluded that **nickel compounds are carcinogenic to humans; metallic nickel is possibly carcinogenic to humans.**

3   CHROMIUM

Epidemiological Studies on Cancer[1]

Clinical observations from Germany in the 1930's raised the suspicion that workers in chromate production plants were at elevated risk to lung cancer, and in the beginning of the 1950's several epidemiological investigations mainly in the US demonstrated the presence of such a risk. Similar studies with similar results have also been performed in the Federal Republic of Germany, Italy, Japan, and UK. The chromium species to which the workers are exposed in chromate production include both trivalent chromium species from the raw materials, and hexavalent chromium species, such as sodium chromates, in the process and products.

Similarly, epidemiological studies in the FRG, France, the Netherlands, Norway, the UK and the USA have consistently shown that workers in chromium pigment industry are at an elevated risk for lung cancer. They have been exposed to soluble chromates in the starting material (alkaline chromates, mainly sodium chromate and dichromate), the rather insoluble hexavalent chromium pigments (barium, lead, molybdenum, zinc, and/or strontium chromates, chromic oxide), and also to some intermediates in the process. It has seldom been possible to study groups of people that have been exclusively engaged in the production of one single chromium pigment. However, from the few existing studies it seems that lung cancer risk is definitely elevated in the production of zinc chromates; in the only available small study on workers in lead chromate production, the overall risk of lung cancer was not elevated, but a significant elevated risk was observed in a subgroup who had previously experienced lead poisoning.

In one large and three small studies among chromium platers, the risk for lung cancer was elevated, and a similar finding was reported for a group of workers in chromium plating and die casting industries in the USA. Workers in this industry are exposed to soluble chromium(VI) compounds, mainly to chromic acid as a mist, but may also be exposed to nickel, since many of these plants also carry out nickel plating. However, in the large British study the lung cancer risk was associated with work experience at chrome baths, but not to that at nickel baths, indicating that chromium probably was the major factor in determining the lung cancer risk.

In two studies among workers in ferrochromium industry, an increased risk for lung cancer was elevated, while in a third no such risk was observed. In these ferrochromium plants workers were exposed to high concentrations of both hexavalent and trivalent chromium compounds, and in one of the two positive studies, also to polycyclic aromatic hydrocarbons.

Cases of sinonasal cancer were reported in epidemiological studies among chromate production, chromate pigment production, and chromium plating. Although no formal statistical analysis could be performed for this rare tumour in these studies, it is quite clear that there was an excess risk for this cancer. Other types of cancer, except for the lung and sinonasal cancer, have not shown consistent associations with exposure to chromium compounds.

No informative epidemiological studies on cancer were available on people exposed solely to trivalent or metallic chromium.

Evaluation. The IARC working group concluded that there is **sufficient evidence** in humans for the carcinogenicity of chromium(VI) compounds as encountered in the chromate production, chromium pigment production and chromium plating industries, and that there is **inadequate evidence** in humans for the carcinogenicity of metallic chromium and of chromium(III) compounds.

Experimental studies on cancer

Metallic chromium. Several old studies are available on the carcinogenicity of metallic chromium, using intratracheal, intramuscular, intrafemoral, intrapleural, intraperitoneal or intravenous routes of administration. None of them have indicated carcinogenic potential, but all of the studies suffer from different limitations of design, reporting, or survival, and therefore do not demonstrate lack of carcinogenicity.

Trivalent chromium compounds. The carcinogenicity of **chromic acetate**, **chromic oxide**, **chloride**, **sulfate**, **chromic tan**, and **chromite ore** have been investigated using oral, intrapleural, intramuscular or intraperitoneal or intrafemoral routes of administration, without evidence of carcinogenicity. These studies suffer from various limitations; however, chromic oxide, chromic chloride, chrome tan and chromite ore were negative even in carefully planned and executed studies with rats using intrabronchial implantation as the route of administration. In these studies a clear cut carcinogenic response was observed after exposure to several hexavalent chromium species (Table 3)[9,10].

Hexavalent chromium compounds. After inhalation exposure to **chromic acid** mist, a few pulmonary adenomas and adenocarcinomas, and nasal adenomas were observed in mice; in two experiments using intrabronchial pellet administration, similarly a few lung tumours were observed (Table 3). When rats were exposed to three different concentrations of **sodium dichromate** by inhalation, a low frequency of pulmonary tumours (2 adenomas and 1 carcinoma) were observed in the group with highest exposure in one study. In another inhalation study no tumours were observed. A dose-dependent increase in malignant pulmonary tumours was observed in rats after multiple intratracheal instillations of sodium dichromate, while only 1 tumour was observed after intrabronchial pellet administration in two experiments with altogether 200 animals (Table 3).

Sodium chromate did not induce lung tumours after intrabronchial pellet administration (Table 3).

A small number of adenomas, but no carcinomas, in mice, and two malignant tumours in rats, were observed after inhalation exposure to **calcium chromate** dust. A dose-dependent increase in pulmonary adenomas and carcinomas was observed in rats after repeated intratracheal instillation of calcium chromate; in three studies pulmonary tumours were observed after intrabronchial administration of calcium chromate-containing pellets. Local tumours were induced by intramuscular and intrapleural administration of calcium chromate.

Different **zinc chromates** induced pulmonary tumours after intrabronchial administration (Table 3), and local tumours were observed after subcutaneous, intramuscular and intrapleural administrations.

Table 3. Pulmonary carcinogenic response after exposure to different chromium species by intrabronchial implantation[9,10]. Numbers of animals with malignant pulmonary tumours over the total number of animals per group have been given.

Chromium species administered	Tumours
Chromium(III) chloride hexahydrate	0/100
Chromic(III) oxide	0/100
Chromite(III) ore	0/100
High silica chrome(III) ore	0/101
Chrome tan (basic Cr(III) sulfate)	0/100
Chromic (VI) acid	1/100
Chromic (VI) acid	2/100
Sodium dichromate	0/100
Sodium dichromate	1/100
Sodium chromate	0/100
Calcium chromate	8/100
Calcium chromate	25/100
Zinc potassium chromate	3/100
Zinc chromate IW	5/100
Zinc chromate ("Norge")	3/100
Zinc tetroxychromate	1/100
Lead chromate	1/98
Primrose chrome yellow (Pb-chromate)	1/100
Molybdate chrome orange (Pb-chromate)	1/100
Light chrome yellow (Pb-chromate)	0/100
LD chrome yellow (Pb-chromate)	1/100
Medium chrome yellow (Pb-chromate)	1/100
Silica encapsulated medium chrome yellow (Pb-chromate)	0/100
Barium chromate	0/100
Strontium chromate (54.1% CrO_4)	43/100
Strontium chromate (24.3% CrO_4)	62/99
Control	0/400

A large number of different **lead chromates** were tested using the intrabronchial pellet administration (Table 3), and altogether 5 malignant pulmonary tumours were observed in 698 animals. The frequency thus was rather low, but on the other hand, no such tumours were observed in 400 contemporary controls in two separate experiments. Lead chromates have also caused local sarcomas after subcutaneous and intramuscular injection; in one such study also the frequency of renal tumours was increased.

Barium chromate did not induce lung tumours after intrabronchial administration; it did not elicit tumours in three limited studies using intramuscular or intrapleural administration either.

Two different **strontium chromate** pigments induced a high incidence of malignant lung tumours in rats after intrabronchial administration; strontium chromate also induced local sarcomas after intrapleural and intramuscular injection.

Evaluation. The IARC working group concluded that for calcium chromate, zinc chromates, strontium chromate and lead chromates, there is **sufficient evidence,** for chromium trioxide (chromic acid) and sodium dichromate there is **limited evidence,** and for metallic chromium, barium chromate and chromium(III) compounds there is **inadequate evidence** of carcinogenicity in experimental animals.

Other relevant data.

The frequency of chromosomal aberrations was elevated in three studies in chromium plating workers; in four studies of six, the frequency of sister chromatid exchanges was also elevated.

Hexavalent chromium compounds of various solubilities, including ammonium, potassium and sodium dichromate, ammonium, calcium, potassium, sodium, strontium chromate, chromium trioxide, zinc yellow, zinc chromate, lead chromate, barium chromate, and derived pigments such as chromium orange, chromium yellow and molybdenum orange, were consistently active in a very large number of studies covering a wide range of tests for genetic and related effects. Some of the slightly soluble pigments required preliminary dissolution in alkali or acids before the effect could fully be observed.

Chromium(III) compounds were generally inactive in tests for genetic activity, or required orders of magnitude higher concentrations than hexavalent chromium compounds to give positive results. However, they were more active than hexavalent chromium compounds in their reaction with purified DNA, or isolated nuclei. Chromium(VI) compounds penetrate cell membranes much more avidly than do trivalent chromium compounds.

Evaluation

The IARC working group made the evaluation of carcinogenicity of hexavalent chromium compounds as a group, as the epidemiological studies, carcinogenicity studies in animals, and several types of other relevant data support the concept that chromium(VI) ions generated at critical sites in the target cells are responsible for the carcinogenic action observed, and concluded that **Chromium(VI) is carcinogenic to humans**, and **metallic chromium and chromium(III) compounds are not classifiable as to their carcinogenicity**.

3 REFERENCES

1. 'IARC Monographs on the evaluation of carcinogenic risks to humans. Chromium, nickel and welding.' International Agency for Research on Cancer, Lyons, France, 1990, in press.
2. Chief Inspector of Factories, 'Annual Report of the Chief Inspector of Factories for the Year 1932, HMSO, London, 1933, p. 103
3. R. Doll, Brit. J. Ind. Med., 1958, 15, 217.
4. J.G. Morgan, Brit. J. Ind. Med., 1958, 15, 224.
5. 'IARC Monographs on the evaluation of carcinogenic risk of chemicals to man. Cadmium, nickel, some epoxides, miscellaneous industrial chemicals and general considerations on volatile anaesthetics. Vol. 11.' International Agency for Research on Cancer, Lyons, France, 1976
6. 'IARC Monographs on the evaluation of carcinogenic risk of chemicals to humans. Supplement No. 4. Chemicals, industrial processes and industries associated with cancer in humans (IARC Monographs Volumes 1 to 29).' International Agency for Research on Cancer, Lyons, France, 1982
7. 'IARC Monographs on the evaluation of carcinogenic risks to humans. Supplement No. 7. Overall evaluations of carcinogenicity: An updating of IARC Monographs Volumes 1 to 42. Supplement 7.' International Agency for Research on Cancer, Lyons, France, 1987
8. International Committee on Nickel Carcinogenesis in Man, Scand. J. Work Environ. Health, 1990, 16, 1.
9. L.S. Levy, P.A. Martin and P.L. Bidstrup, Brit. J. Ind. Med., 1986, 43, 243.
10. L.S. Levy and S. Venitt, Carcinogenesis, 1986, 7, 831.

Teratogenicity of Ni^{2+} in *Xenopus Laevis*

S. M. Hopfer[1], M. C. Plowman[1], K. R. Sweeney[2], J. A. Bantle[3], and F. W. Sunderman, Jr.[1]

[1] DEPARTMENTS OF LABORATORY MEDICINE AND PHARMACOLOGY, SCHOOL OF MEDICINE, UNIVERSITY OF CONNECTICUT, FARMINGTON, CT 06030;
[2] SCHOOL OF PHARMACY, UNIVERSITY OF CONNECTICUT, STORRS, CT O6268; AND
[3] DEPARTMENT OF ZOOLOGY, OKLAHOMA STATE UNIVERSITY, STILLWATER, OK 74078, USA

1 INTRODUCTION

This chapter is an extended abstract of a study by Hopfer et al[1] in which the teratogenicity of Ni^{2+} was assayed by the FETAX (Frog Embryo Teratogenesis Assay: Xenopus) procedure. This technique, developed by Dumont et al[2] and standardized by investigations in Bantle's laboratory,[3-5] has been validated as a screening test for teratogenic hazards from chemical agents.[6-8] The FETAX assay has been applied to numerous organic compounds, drugs, and environmental samples.[9-12]

2 MATERIALS AND METHODS

Experimental Animals and Test Chemical

Mature *Xenopus laevis* (Xenopus I, Inc., Ann Arbor, MI) were housed at 20 $\pm$ 1° C in polycarbonate aquaria. The frogs were fed three times per week, once with pelleted frog chow and twice with a mixture of beef heart and lung. NiCl$_2$, 99.999 % pure, was purchased from Ventron Corp., Danvers, MA, USA.

Ovulation

Three days before each assay, an adult female was primed by an injection of pregnant mare serum (0.1 mL) into the dorsal lymph sac. On the evening before the assay, the female was given an injection of human chorionic gonatotropin (600 IU) into the dorsal lymph sac. The female was kept overnight at 16° C. Next morning, the female was firmly squeezed so that 300 to 400 eggs were expelled into a plastic Petri dish. The eggs were promptly fertilized by adding a suspension of *Xenopus* sperm. The process was repeated thrice, so that 900 to 1.200 eggs from each female were harvested for fertilization.

Fertilization and Development to the Blastula Stage

A testicle was excised from an adult *Xenopus* male and placed in 5 mL of Tris phosphate buffer (pH 7.6, 4° C). One third of the testicle was gently minced in a polypropylene microfuge tube that contained 1 mL of FETAX medium[3]. The FETAX medium was adjusted to ph 6.8 to avoid precipitation of $Ni(OH)_2$. The sperm suspension was pipetted over the eggs and 45 sec was allowed for sperm attachment, before FETAX medium was added to cover the eggs in the Petri dish. After 20 min, the eggs were dejellied by swirling for 3 min in FETAX medium that contained L-cysteine HCl (0.13 mol/L) adjusted to pH 8.0 with dilute NaOH solution. The L-cysteine HCl was removed by washing the eggs four times with FETAX medium, transferring them to a clean Petri dish, and washing them four more times with FETAX medium. The developing embryos were kept in an incubator at 23 $\pm$ 1° C until the FETAX assay began at 5 h post-fertilization, by which time the embryos had reached the large-cell blastula stage[13]. Only normally cleaving embryos were selected for the FETAX assay.

FETAX Assay

The standard FETAX procedure was performed according to Dumont et al[2] and Dawson and Bantle[3], with the following specifications. Each assay comprised 24 to 30 Petri dishes that contained ~22 *Xenopus* embryos. Quadruplicate Petri dishes contained control embryos (~88/test) in FETAX medium. Ten to 13 sets of duplicate Petri dishes contained test embryos (~44/Ni level) in FETAX test media with graded Ni^{2+} concentrations. The assay was repeated 7 times and the following 22 concentrations of Ni^{2+} were tested in at least two assays: 0.1, 0.3, 1.0, 1.8, 2.7, 3.0, 3.6, 4.5, 5.6, 10, 30, 100, 180, 270, 300, 360, 450, 540, 560, 1,000, 1,800 and 3,000 mol/L. The FETAX medium contained < 0.05 mol Ni/L, based on EAAS analyses[14]. The Petri dishes were kept at 23 $\pm$ 1° C; the media were changed and dead embryos were removed at 29, 53 and 75 h post-fertilization. At 101 h post-fertilization, surviving tadpoles were counted, fixed in formalin (3%, v/v), and examined with a dissecting microscope to determine their developmental stages, malformations, and head-to-tail lengths[2,3,13].

Modified FETAX Assay

To determine when *Xenopus* embryos were most susceptible to Ni^{2+}teratogenesis the following modification was used in four FETAX assays: Embryos in sets of duplicate Petri dishes (~22 embryos/dish) were exposed during four 24-h intervals post-fertilization (*ie.*, 5 - 29 h, 29 - 53 h, 53 - 75 h or 75 - 101 h) to test medium that contained Ni^{2+} (30 mol/L). At other times, the embryos were exposed to FETAX medium without added Ni^{2+}. At 101 h post-fertilization, the assays were terminated and surviving tadpoles were scored by the usual procedure.

Statistical Analyses

Values for LC_{10}, LC_{50}, and LC_{90} (mortality) and EC_{10}, EC_{50} and EC_{90} (malformation) were computed by the Litchfield-Wilcoxson test[15] using an iterative, least-squares computer program, 'PCNONLIN'[16]. Values for Teratogenic Index (TI=LC_{50}/EC_{50}) and Minimum Concentration to Inhibit Growth (MCIG) were computed as previously described[2,7]. Standard deviations (SD), standard errors (SE), linear regression analysis, Spearman's correlation coefficient (r), ANOVA, and Student's t test were computed by standard methods[17].

3 RESULTS

The standard FETAX assay of Ni^{2+} was repeated seven times with similar results. In control embryos, survival at 101 h post-fertilization was consistently $\geq$ 95 % and the incidence of malformations was $\leq$ 7 %. In Ni^{2+} -exposed embryos, the embryolethal concentrations of Ni^{2+} were as follows: LC_{10} = 224 (SE $\pm$ 11) mol/L LC_{50} = 365 (SE $\pm$ 9) mol/L, and LC_{90} = 595 (SE $\pm$ 36) mol/L. The corresponding teratogenic concentrations of Ni^{2+} were as follows: EC_{10} = 1.44 (SE $\pm$ 0.08) mol/L, EC_{50} = 2.49 (SE $\pm$ 0.08) mol/L, and EC_{90} = 4.30 (SE $\pm$ 0.24) mol/L. The Teratogenic Index (TI = LC_{50}/EC_{50}) for Ni^{2+} was 147 (SE $\pm$ 5), far exceeding the TI of 1.5 that is considered the threshold level for positive teratogenicity in the FETAX assay[5].

The following anomalies were seen at graded Ni^{2+} - exposures:

Ni^{2+}, 3 mol/L: The tip of the tail was bent downward in many embryos. Gut coiling was impaired and craniofacial anomalies were occasionally seen. Eyes tended to be small, misshapen, and hypopigmented, and the choroid fissure oft-times failed to fuse. The dorsal fin generally projected upward from the vertebrae.

Ni^{2+}, 30 mol/L: The tip of the tail was usually kinked downward and craniofacial anomalies were frequent. Gut coiling was incomplete and the heart was variably enlarged, projecting forward (cardioptosis). The eyes commonly showed hypopigmentation and failure of the choroid fissure to fuse. The dorsal and ventral fins extended broadly from the vertebrae.

Ni^{2+}, 100 mol/L: The embryos were all malformed and stunted growth was obvious. Anomalies of the head, facial, and axial skeleton were prevalent, including frequent vertebral fusions and hunchback deformity. The eyes were generally misshapen and sometimes bizarrely deformed. Gut coiling was further reduced. Cardiomegaly, cardioptosis, and fin ruffling were prominent.

Ni^{2+}, 300 mol/L: The embryos were extremely deformed and stunted. The tail generally bent upward, although its tip was kinked downward. Severe facial malformations were common, including cleft lip and palate, midfacial hypoplasia, and upward displacement of the nares. Cut coiling was limited to a few large loops. The eyes were malformed, with open choroid fissure, scleral herniation, depigmentation, microphthalmia, and sometimes anophthalmia. Fin ruffling and expansion were severe and dermal blisters or blebs formed over the surface of the body.

Other abnormalities, not categorized as malformations, became more prominent with increasing Ni^{2+} concentrations, such as stunted growth, effusions or hemorrhages into the coelomic cavities, and dermal hypopigmentation. The Minimum Concentration to Inhibit Growth (MCIG) for Ni^{2+} in the FETAX assay was 5.6 mol/L.

In modified FETAX assay, *Xenopus* embryos were exposed to FETAX test medium that contained Ni^{2+} (30 mol/L) during specific 24 h periods, as follows: Group A, 5-29 h; Group B, 29-53 h; Group C, 53-75 h; and Group D, 75-101 h. At other times, the embryos were kept in FETAX medium without added Ni^{2+}. When the assays were terminated at 101 h post-fertilization, the proportions of malformed embryos among the survivors in the respective groups were as follows: Group A, 32/123 (26 %); Group B, 112/122 (92 %); Group C, 117/117 (100 %), and Group D, 24/117 (21 %) (p<0.01 by ANOVA). Thus, *Xenopus* embryos are most susceptible to Ni^{2+}-induced malformations on the second and third days of life. The pattern of Ni^{2+}-induced malformations was affected by the timing of the exposures, since facial, cardiac, and intestinal anomalies were more common in Group C than in Group B ($p<0.05$), while ocular or skeletal anomalies were almost equally common in the two groups.

4 DISCUSSION

Previous studies showed that Ni^{2+} compounds are embryotoxic for the mouse,[18,19] rat,[20-24] hamster,[25] chick,[26] and sea urchin[27]. Teratogenic responses to Ni^{2+} - exposures were reported in mice,[18,28] chicks,[29] and sea urchins.[27] In addition, fetal malformations were observed after exposures of pregnant rats or hamsters to $Ni(CO)_4$,[30-32] which undergoes oxidation in vivo to Ni^{2+}.[33] The present study[1] showed that Ni^{2+} is a potent teratogen for Xenopus, inducing malformations of the eyes, skeleton, intestine, face, heart, and integumen. The Teratogenic Index (TI) of 147 for Ni^{2+} in the FETAX assay was higher than the reported TI values of 4.5 for hydroxyurea[6] and 11.8 for 5-fluorouracil,[3] which are established mammalian teratogens.

Lin et al.[34] have reported that Xenopus embryos possess a 31 kD protein that avidly binds $^{63}Ni^{2+}$ in vitro. The role of the 31 kD protein in the uptake of Ni^{2+} by Xenopus embryos is being investigated in our laboratory. The authors believe that the FETAX assay provides a convenient and standardized system to study the molecular mechanisms of chemical teratogenesis, as well as a practical technique to screen chemical compounds for teratogenic effects.

5 REFERENCES

1. S.M. Hopfer, M.C. Plowman, K.R. Sweeney, J.A. Bantle, F.W. Sunderman Jr, Biol. Trace Elem. Res.(in press).
2. J.N. Dumont, T.W. Schultz, M. Buchanan, G. Kao 'Application of Short-term Bioassays in the Analysis of Complex Environmental Mixtures', M.D. Waters, S.S. Sandhu, J. Lewtas, L. Claxon, N. Chernoff, S. Nesnow, eds., Plenum Press, New York, p 393, 1983.
3. D.A. Dawson and J.A. Blantle, J. Appl. Toxicol., 1987, 7, 237.
4. D.J. Fort, D.A. Dawson, J.A. Bantle, Teratog. Carcinog. Mutagen., 1988, 8, 251.
5. D.J. Fort and J.A. Bantle, Fundam. Appl. Toxicol., 1990, 14, 720.
6. T.D. Sabourin, R.T. Faulk, L.B. Goss, J. Appl. Toxicol., 1985, 5, 227.
7. D.A. Dawson, E.F. Stebler, S.L. Burks, J.A. Bantle, Environ. Toxicol. Chem., 1988, 7, 27.

8. J.A. Bantle, D.F. Fort, B.L. James, Hydrobiologia 1989, 188, 577.
9. C.L. Courchesne, J.A. Bantle, Teratog. Carcinog. Mutagen., 1985, 5, 177.
10. D.A. Dawson, J.A. Bantle, Teratology, 1987, 35, 221.
11. D.A. Dawson, D.J. Fort, G.J. Smith, D.L. Newell, J.A. Bantle, Teratog. Carcinog. Mutagen., 1988, 8, 32.
12 D.A. Dawson, D.J. Fort, D.L. Newell, J.A. Bantle, Drug. Chem. Toxicol., 1989, 12, 67.
13. P.D. Nieuwkoop, J.Faber, 'Normal Table of Xenopus laevis (Daudin),'2nd edition, Elsevier/North Holland Biomedical Press, Amsterdam, 1967.
14. F.W. Sunderman Jr., S.M. Hopfer, M.C. Crisostomo, Meth. Enzymol., 1988, 158, 382.
15. J.T. Litchfield, F. Wilcoxson, J. Pharmacol. Exp. Ther., 1949, 96, 99.
16. C.M. Metzler, D.L. Weiner, Am. Statistician. 1986, 40, 1.
17. L.Sachs, 'Applied Statistics,'Springer-Verlag, New York, 1984.
18. C.-C. Lu, N. Matsumoto, S. Iijima, Teratology 1979, 19, 137.
19. R. Storeng, J. Jonsen, Toxicology, 1980, 17, 183.
20. H.A. Schroeder, M. Mitchener, Arch. Environ. Health, 1971, 23, 102.
21. A.M. Ambrose, P.S. Larson, J.F. Borzelleca, G.F. Hennigar Jr., J. Food Sci. Tech.,1976, 13, 181.
22. F.W. Sunderman Jr., S.K. Shen, J.M. Mitchell, P.R. Alpass, I.Damjanov, Toxicol. Appl. Pharmacol., 1978, 43, 381.
23. V.G. Nadeenko, V. Lenchenko, T.A. Archipenko, S.P. Saichenko, Gig. Sanit., 1979, 6, 86.
24. C.H. Weischer, W. Kordel, D. Hochrainer, Zbl. Bact. Hyg. B, 1980, 171, 336.
25. V.H. Ferm, Adv. Teratol.,1972, 5, 51.
26 L.P. Ridgeway, D.A. Karnovsky, Ann. N. Y. Acad. Sci.,1952, 55, 203.
27. H. Timourian, G.Watchmaker, J. Exp. Zool., 1972, 182, 379.
28. R.Storeng, J. Jonsen, Toxicology, 1981, 20, 45.
29. S.H. Gilani, M. Marano, Arch. Environ. Contam. Toxicol., 1980, 9, 17.
30. F.W. Sunderman Jr., P.R. Allpass, J.M. Mitchell, R.C. Baselt, D.M. Albert, Science, 1979, 203, 550.
31. F.W. Sunderman Jr., S.K. Shen, M.C. Reid, P.R. Allpass, Teratog. Carcinog. Mutagen., 1980, 1, 223.
32. F.W. Sunderman Jr., M.C. Reid, S.K. Shen, C.B. Kevorkian, Reproductive and Developmental Toxicology of Metals, T.W. Clarkson, G.F. Nordberg, P.R. Sager, eds., Plenum Press, New York, 1983, p 399.
33. F.W. Sunderman Jr., C.E. Selin, Toxicol. Appl. Pharmacol., 1968, 12, 207.

34. S.-M. Lin, S.M. Hopfer, S.M. Brennan, and F.W. Sunderman Jr., Res. Commun. Chem. Pathol. Pharmacol., 1989, 65, 275.

Mechanisms of Action of Trace Elements

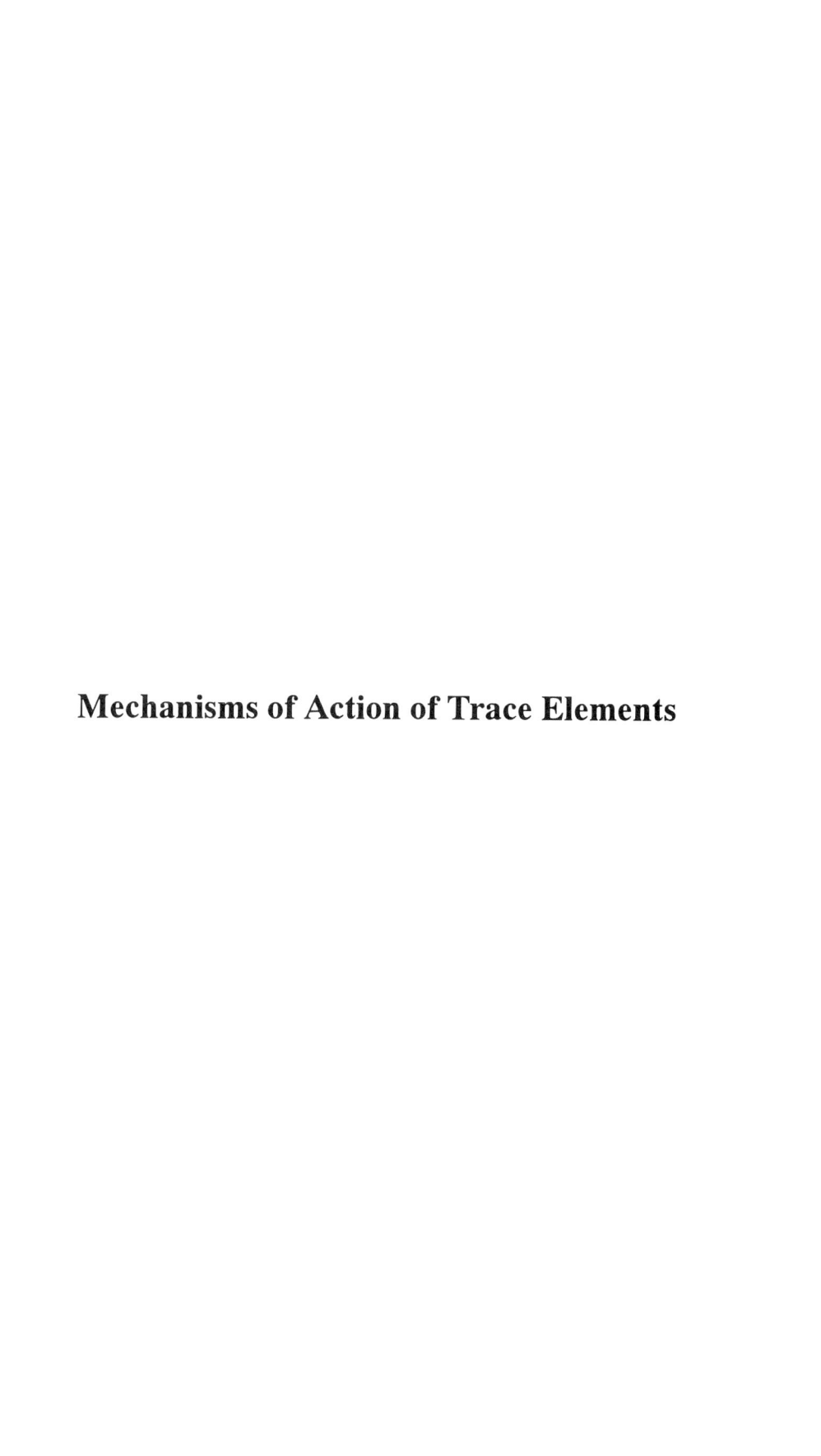

The Significance of Target Cells for a Model of Uptake and Biological Transformation of αNi_3S_2

H. F. Hildebrand*, P. Shirali*, F. Z. Arrouijal*, A. M. Decaestecker*, and R. Martinez**

* INSTITUT DE MÉDECINE DU TRAVAIL, FACULTÉ DE MÉDECINE, 1, PLACE DE VERDUN, F. 59045 LILLE CÉDEX, FRANCE
** CNRS UA 234, UNIVERSITÉ DE LILLE I, F. 59655 VILLENEUVE D'ASCQ CÉDEX, FRANCE

1 INTRODUCTION

In a recent review Sunderman[1] underlined that one of the major determinants of carcinogenic and toxic effects of nickel compounds is their cellular bioavailability, *i.e.* the ability of nickel to enter target cells and to release nickel ions which interact with cellular constituents and molecules. This implies different mechanisms of cellular uptake, biological transformation and cellular transport. Nickel subsulfide, αNi_3S_2, is considered to belong to the most carcinogenic nickel compounds as shown in experimental animals.[2] Its toxic, carcinogenic and mutagenic effects have also been demonstrated in numerous *in vitro* bioassays.[3] Different cell types have been used for these investigations without any special care for whether the cell type used can be considered as target cell or not. The "target cell" concept, however, is certainly important, as mentioned above, for any study with respect to the cellular bioavailability of nickel compounds. Thus the present study will deal with the uptake, incorporation and biological transformation of Ni_3S_2 and its subsequent binding to constituents of different cell types which are either considered as target cells in human and animal pathology or are frequently used in mutagenicity tests.

2 MATERIAL AND METHODS

Nickel subsulfide, αNi_3S_2, (purity 99.5 %, particle size 1.4 µm) was provided by INCO Ltd, Toronto, Ontario, Canada.
Seven different cell types were used for the present study: human embryonic epithelial lung cells (L132 cell line); guinea pig alveolar macrophages (GPAM) obtained from Hartley albinos by bronchoalveolar lavage; Wistar rat lymphocytes (RL), *in vivo* and *in vitro*; human lymphocytes from sensitized (HLS) and unsensitized (HLU) persons to nickel, CHO cells; and V79 cells. All cells

were exposed to 50 µmol/L Ni$_3$S$_2$ during 3 days. RL, CHO, L132 were cultured in MEM 0011 medium (Eurobio), HLU and HLS in RPMI 1640 medium (Flow), GPAM in MEM 2011 medium (Eurobio), and V79 in H21 medium (GIBCO). All culture media were supplemented with 5 % foetal calf serum. In addition, Ni$_3$S$_2$ was treated at the same concentrations and under the same culture conditions with MEM 0011 medium.

In vivo incorporation in RL was studied by i.v. injections of 80 mg Ni$_3$S$_2$ per rat. The incubation time was also 3 days.

For ultrastructural investigations cell pellets were prepared by light centrifugation (300 g) and fixed for 20 min in 2.5 % glutaraldehyde in the respectice culture medium without foetal calf serum. After two washes in the medium, the cell pellets were postfixed for 20 min in 1 % OsO$_4$ in sodium phosphate buffer (pH 7.2) or sodium cacodylate buffer (pH 7.2) for control. After dehydration in ethanol, the cell pellets were embedded in Epicote. Unstained sections were examined with with Philips EM300 and ZEISS EM 10CR electron microscopes. Electron microprobe analyses by X-ray energy dispersive spectrometry (EDS) were performed on unstained sections placed on Pioloform F coated titanium or carbon coated nylon grids. Elemental determinations were carried out with a Jeol 200CX electron microscope connected to a Link QX200 analytical system.

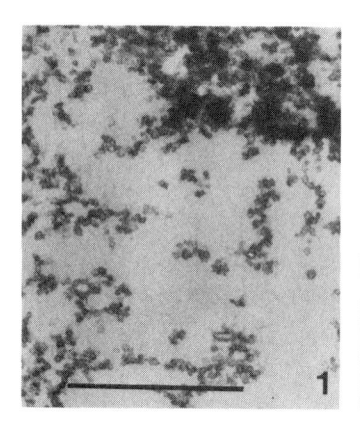

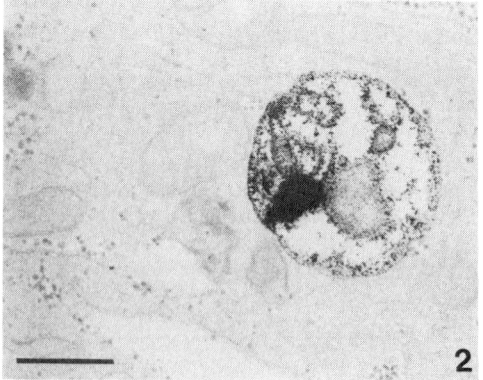

Fig. 1
Extracellular degradation of Ni$_3$S$_2$ to tiny particles.
Bar: 1 µm

Fig. 2
Ni$_3$S$_2$ transformation in a phagocytic vacuole of a L132 cell containing a crystal fragment and tiny particles bound to the vacuolar and lysosomal membranes
Bar: 0.5 µm

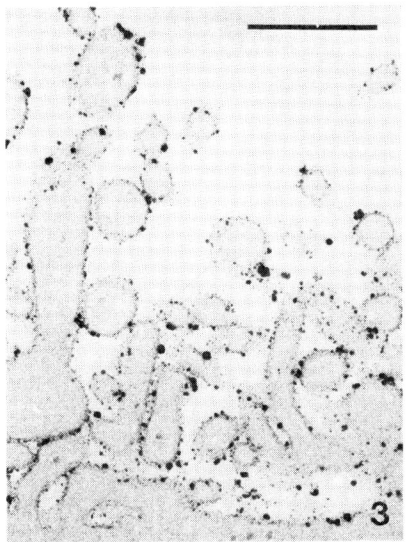

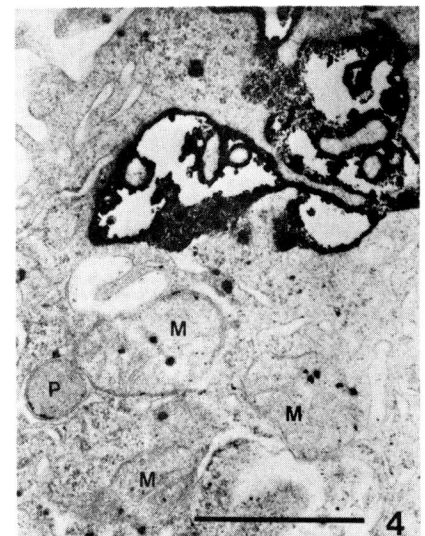

Fig. 3
L132 cell presenting a high amount of microvilli strongly labelled with tiny particles on the outer layer of the cell membrane
Bar: 0.5 μm

Fig. 4
GPAM presenting a phagocytic vacuole with lysosomal structures. Cytoplasmic tiny particles are preferentially bound to mitochondria (M) and peroxisomes (P)
Bar: 1 μm

3 RESULTS AND DISCUSSION

Ultrastructural Investigations

The ultrastructural studies followed by EDS analyses were carried out on Ni_3S_2 incubated alone under culture conditions and on three groups of cells: (i) pulmonary cells (L132, GPAM), probably target cells in pulmonary pathogenesis; (ii) lymphocytes (RL, HLU, HLS), target cells for immunological reactions; and (iii) on two cell types (V79, CHO), frequently used for mutagenicity tests.

Culture Media

Ni_3S_2 Crystals submitted to culture conditions are broken into smaller fragments which are further transformed to tiny particles with an average size of 10 to 30 nm arranged in strings or chains (Fig. 1). These arrangements are probably due to a complexation of the degradation product with fibrillar macromolecules. They can be compared to those appearing in extracellular spaces of L132 cells cultured in the presence of Ni_3S_2.[4]

182   *Trace Elements in Health and Disease*

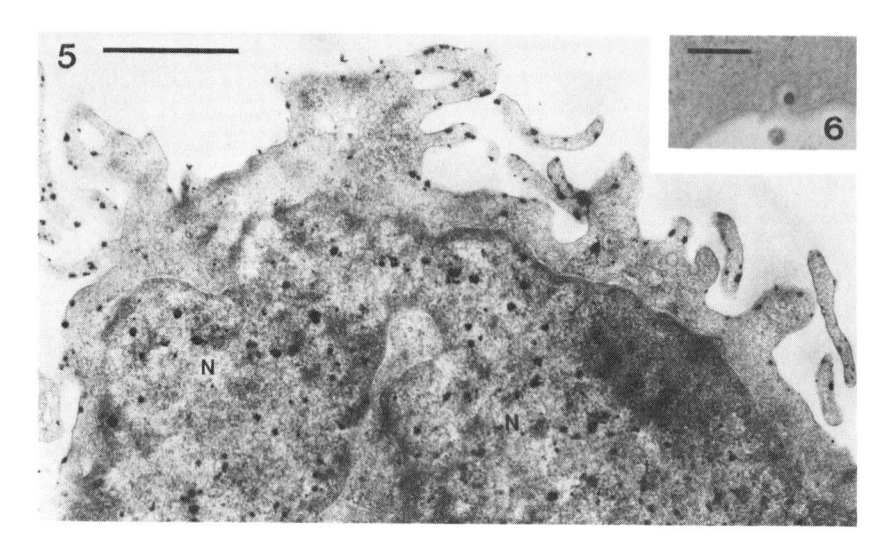

Fig. 5
Tiny particles bound to the inner layer of cell membranes and the euchromatinic part of nucleus (N) in a GPAM
Bar: 1 µm

Fig. 6
Endocytosis process of a small round particle in a GPAM
Bar: 0.25 µm

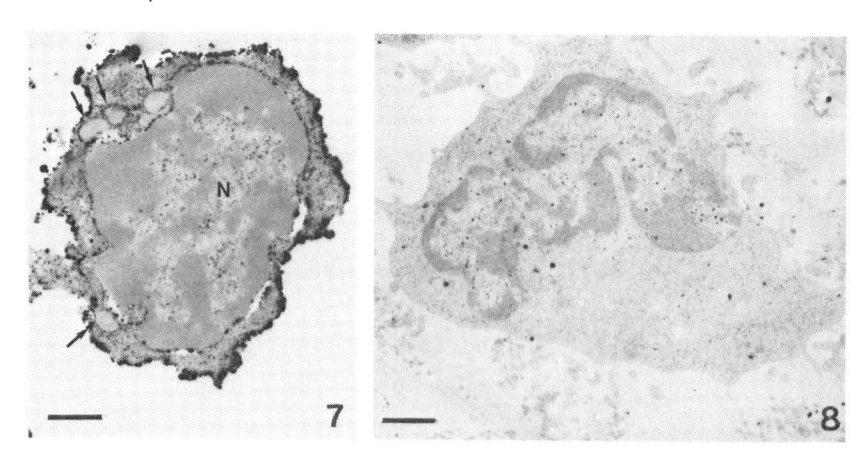

Fig. 7
Tiny particles bound to rat lymphocytes incubated *in vitro* on the outer layer of cell membrane, on mitochondria (arrows), nuclear membranes, and the euchromatine in the nucleus (N)
Bar: 1 µm

Fig. 8
Ni_3S_2 degradation in rat lymphocytes incubated *in vivo*. The labelling of cell structures is similar to that observed in lymphocytes incubated *in vitro*, but less important. The preferential binding of particles in euchromatine is evident
Bar: 1 µm

L132 Cells

In L132 cells two major events are observed. Phagocytosis of crystals is common: cells generally exhibit several vacuoles with crystals in a degradation process to tiny particles with an average size of 10 nm covering the phagocytic vacuole and bound to lysosomal membranes (Fig. 2). The second event is the extracellular degradation of crystals and the binding of particles on the outer layer of cell membrane and microvilli in a particular dense disposition (Fig. 3). These particles are rarely observed on other cellular constituents and never on nuclear structures.[4]

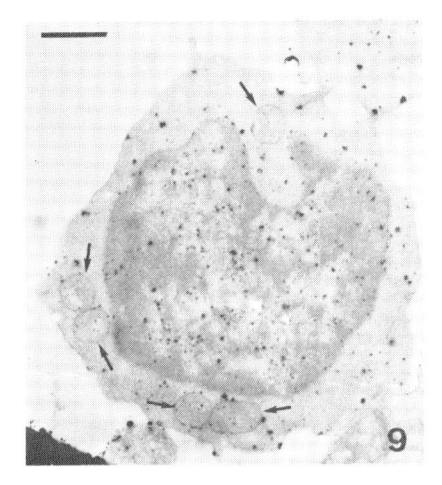

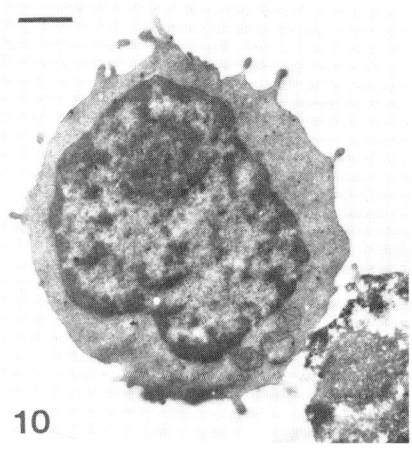

Fig. 9
Ni_3S_2 incorporation in a human lymphocyte from a Ni-sensitized person (HLS). Euchromatine and mitochondria (arrows) are strongly labelled by tiny particles
Bar: 1 µm

Fig.10
Ni_3S_2 incorporation in a human lymphocyte from an unsensitized person (HLU). Only very few particles can be observed
Bar: 1 µm

Alveolar Macrophages

In GPAMs we observe an identical phagocytic degradation with subsequent binding of particles to phagocytic and lysosomal membranes (Fig. 4). We have also noted a quantitatively important binding of particles to cellular membranes, which is different from that described for L132 cells. In GPAMs one observes these particles on the outer layer of the cell membrane after an exposure of 24 to 48 h and on the inner layer (Fig. 5) after an exposure of 48 to 72 h.[5] This observation indicates additional cellular uptake by transmembranous passage. We also have often seen round particles entering the cell by endocytosis (Fig. 6). The essential difference between L132 cells and GPAMs is the presence of particles in GPAMs on other cell structures such as endoplasmic reticulum, mitochondria and peroxisomes (Fig. 4) and in particular on the euchromatinic part of nuclei (Fig. 5).[5]

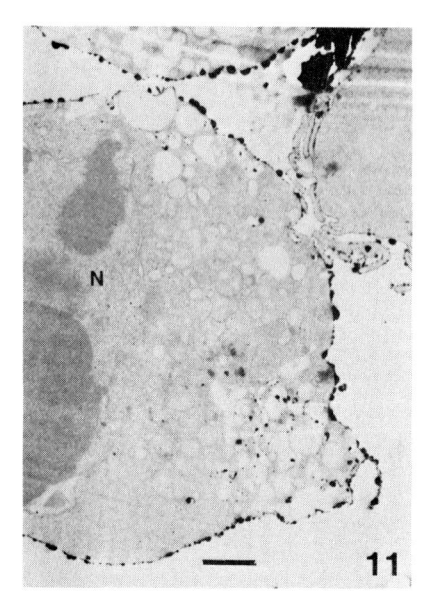

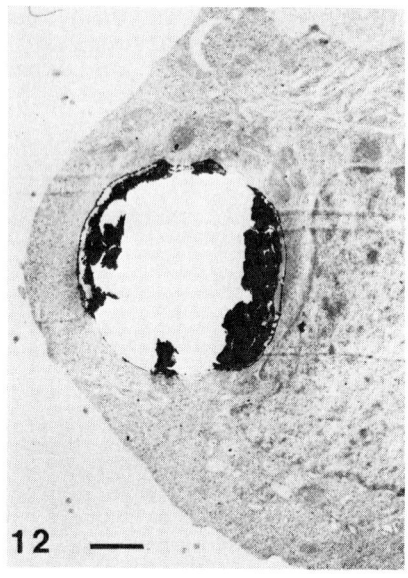

Fig. 11
V79 cell displaying tiny particles on the cell membrane and in some phagocytic vacuoles. No other cell structures are labelled.
N=nucleus
Bar: 1 μm

Fig. 12
The only event observed in CHO cells is phagocytosis of crystals with a slight degradation to particles bound to the vacuolar membrane
Bar: 1 μm

Rat Lymphocytes

In rat lymphocytes we obtained similar results after *in vitro*[6] (Fig. 7) and *in vivo* (Fig. 8) incubation. We also find tiny particles on all cell organelles and in the euchromatinic part of nuclei. The binding of particles to cell and nuclear membranes is less marked after *in vivo* than after *in vitro* incubations. This observation clearly shows that *in vivo* and *in vitro* incubations give nearly identical results which may validate the *in vitro* experiments at least for this cell type.

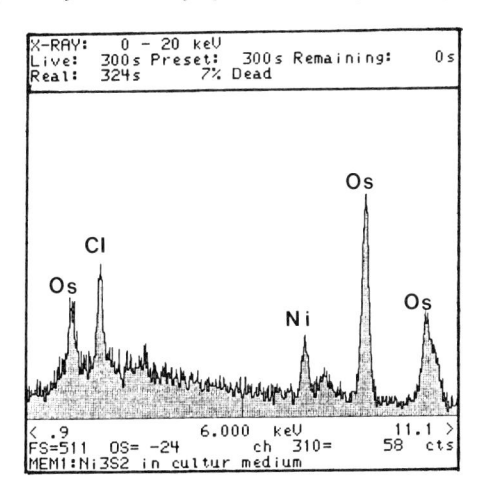

Fig. 13 Typical EDS diagram of extracellular particles. Note the absence of sulfur and the presence of chloride. This diagram also shows the typical distribution of the osmium peaks

Human Lymphocytes

Human Lymphocytes of sensitized persons (HLS) showed identical reactions to Ni_3S_2. Particles are concentrated in particular on mitochondria, endoplasmic reticulum and euchromatine (Fig. 9). In HLUs, however, we could detect only very few particles bound to cellular structures (Fig. 10). We never observed phagocytosis in RLs or in HLU's, but frequently in HLUs. Endocytosis of tiny particles could also be seen in lymphocytes, except in HLUs. Because of the low frequency of particles, this result cannot be taken to demonstrate absence of uptake of particles by endocytosis in these cells.

The binding of particles to cell organelles confirms our previous results about nickel retention in lung cells *in vivo* after i.p. injections of [63]$NiCl_2$ in mice.[7] In that study we demonstrated that the microsomal and mitochondrial subcellular fractions of lung tissue are the target cell fractions of nickel incorporation.

A particularly interesting result is the difference of incorporation in human lymphocytes. Although HLS's show a strong uptake of tiny particles in contrast to HLUs, chromosomal aberrations are significantly more frequent in HLUs than in HLS's.[8] At present we have no other plausible explanation for these apparently contradictory results than that HLS's have special receptors scavenging Ni_3S_2 metabolites, the mutagenic potency of which becomes smaller.

V79 cells

Uptake of Ni_3S_2 by V79 Cells can be compared to its incorporation into L132 cells, although only tiny particles are phagocytized. They also enter the cell by endocytosis (Fig. 11). Furthermore, the particles are observed on the outer layer of cell membranes, but not on other organelles or in the nuclei. Since Ni_3S_2 is also negative in the HPRT test for mutagenicity in these cells,[9] their significance as target cells remains uncertain.

Cho cells

In Cho cells, we observed only phagocytosis of Ni_3S_2 crystals with very little degradation to tiny particles some of which are covering the membrane of the phagocytic vacuole (Fig. 12). No other event, neither endocytosis nor binding of tiny particles to cell membranes, organelles or nuclei has been observed. The cellular pathway proposed by Costa and Heck[10] and Sen and Costa[11] for crystalline nickel sulfides, namely uptake by phagocytosis and interaction with heterochromatine in studies on the same cell type, cannot be confirmed by our observations.

The different events of Ni_3S_2 uptake and the binding sites of tiny particles are summarized in Table 1.

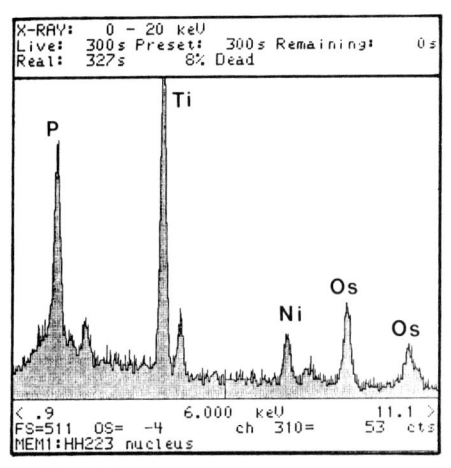

Fig. 14
Typical EDS diagram of tiny particles in euchromatine (here in *in vitro* incubated rat lymphocytes). Note the presence of an important phosphorus peak

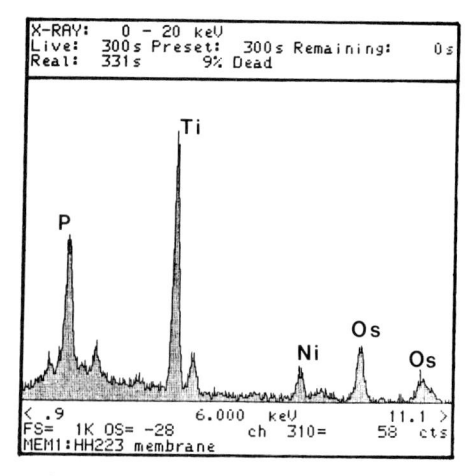

Fig. 15
Typical EDS diagram of tiny particles of a membranous area (here in *in vitro* incubated rat lymphocytes). Note the presence of an important phosphorus peak

Table 1 Ni$_3$S$_2$ Uptake and Binding Sites of Tiny Particles

Cell type	Phagocytosis of crystals	Endocytosis	Cell membrane	Cell organelles	Nuclei Euchromatine
L132[4]	+	+	+	–	–
GPAM[5,12]	+	+	+	+	+
RL in vitro[6]	n.o.	+	+	+	+
RL in vivo	+	+	+	+	+
HLU[6,8]	+	n.o.[xx]	(+)	(+)	(+)
HLS[6,8]	(+)	+	+	+	+
V79[9]	n.o.[x]	+	+	n.o.	–
CHO	+	–	–	–	–

n.o.: not observed, [x] of tiny particles only, [xx] not observed but possible

Energy Despersive Spectrometry (EDS)

EDS analyses of particles generated from Ni$_3$S$_2$ in culture conditions revealed that its degradation to tiny particles is going with a simultanous loss of sulfur via a "Ni$_2$S-like" compound[4] to become a sulfur-free nickel compound (Fig. 13). The same process is detected during degradation in phagocytic vacuoles.

In particles bound to cellular structures, however, one observes the striking emergence of a phosphorus peak. This has been demonstrated in particular for cell membrane bound particles (Fig. 14)[4-6,12] and for those found in the euchromatinic part of nuclei (Fig. 15)[5,6,12]. Similar results of Ni$_3$S$_2$ binding to cellular and phagocytic membranes of other cell types were described by Berry et al.[13] By using another analytical system, these authors did not detect the sulfur-phosphorus shift - which takes place simultanously with the biological transformation of Ni$_3$S$_2$ - that we observed here.

These findings lead us to suggest the formation of an organic Ni/P complex with the phosphate groups of membranous phospholipids or other phospho-transferring molecules.[4-6] First demonstration of the interaction of Ni_3S_2 with aliphatic or fatty acid chains have been given by Shirali et al.[5,12] on L132 cells and GPAMs.

Another Ni/P complex is certainly appearing in the euchromatinic part of nuclei with the phosphate groups of nuclear DNA and/or RNA.[5,6,12] These complexes on cell membranes and especially on euchromatine and for our research team the most important criteria to consider GPAMs, both RLs and HLS's as target cells for pulmonary pathogenesis and immunological reactions respectively, since they present the most widespread incorporation possibilities of all cell types examined.

It has also been shown here that phagocytosis is not the only uptake and not the only pathway in carcinogenesis of Ni_3S_2 or other metal compounds as it has been suggested previously by other authors.[14] These results are more consistent with Sunderman's[2] concept, that the degree of phagocytosis can no longer be considered as a main criterion for the evaluation of carcinogenic activity of any compound. Since there also exists a phagocytic transformation of Ni_3S_2, its carcinogenic effect by this pathway will still have a certain importance. The carcinogenic potency of Ni_3S_2 depends essentially on the way by which it has become bioavailable.

4 REFERENCES

1. F.W. Sunderman Jr, Scand. J. Work Environ. Health, 1989, 15, 1.
2. F.W. Sunderman Jr.:"Nickel in the Human Environment",F.W. Sunderman Jr., ed., Lyon, IARC Sci. Publ., 1984, 53, 127.
3. M. Costa, Environ. Health Perspect., 1989, 81, 73.
4. H.F. Hildebrand, M. Collyn d'Hooghe, P. Shirali, C. Bailly and J.P. Kerckaert, Carcinogenesis, 1990, in press.
5. P. Shirali, H.F. Hildebrand, A.M. Decaestecker, C. Bailly, J.P. Henichart and R. Martinez, Adv. Environ. Sci. Technol., 1990, in press
6. H.F. Hildebrand, A.M. Decaestecker and D. Hetuin, In: Trace Elements in Human Health and Disease", P. Grandjean, ed., Copenhagen, WHO-CEC-EPA Environ. Health Series, 1987,20, 82.
7. M.C. Herlant-Peers, H.F. Hildebrand and J.P. Kerckaert, Carcinogenesis, 1983, 4, 387.
8. F.Z. Arrouijal, H.F. Hildebrand, H. Vo Phi and D. Marzin, 19th Annual Meeting of the European Environm. Mutagenesis Society, Rhodes, Greece, October 21-26, 1989.

9. F.Z. Arrouijal, H.F. Hildebrand, H. Vo Phi and D. Marzin, Mutagenesis, 1990, in press.
10. M. Costa and J.D. Heck, Trends Pharmacol. Sci., 1982, 3, 408.
11. P. Sen and M. Costa, Toxicol. Appl. Pharmacol., 1986, 84, 278.
12. P. Shirali, H.F. Hildebrand, A.M. Decaestecker, C. Bailly and J.P. Henichart, In:"Proceedings of the Intern. Symp. of Industrial Toxicol. "Y. Devillers, ed., Bordeaux-Valenciennes, 1988, pp. 105.
13. J.P. Berry, P. Galle, M.F. Poupon, J. Pot-Deprun, I. Chouroulinkov, J.G. Judde and D. Dewally, In:"Nickel in the Human Environment", F.W. Sunderman Jr. ed., Lyon, IARC Sci. Publ., 1984, 53, 153.
14. M. Costa and H.H. Mollenhauer, Cancer Res., 1980, 40, 2688.

Oxygen Free Radicals, Other Reactive Species and Antioxidants

J. O. Järvisalo

REHABILITATION RESEARCH CENTRE OF THE SOCIAL INSURANCE INSTITUTION, 20720 TURKU, FINLAND

1 INTRODUCTION

During the long era of the oxygen containing atmosphere, life on earth has well adjusted to make best use of the complex physico-chemical properties of oxygen. Examples are the essential role of oxygen in oxidative phosphorylation and in other oxidation processes depending on various respiratory chains, the use of reduced oxygen species for microbicidal purposes by phagocytes and various enzymatic oxidase, oxygenase and peroxidase reactions.

Due to its molecular structure, oxygen is able to accept electrons successively in reduction/oxidation reactions and due to that it may be a mediator of a variety of reactions: reduction of molecular oxygen to two molecules of water is a result of acceptance of four electrons of the molecular oxygen. This full reduction of oxygen occurs in oxidative phosphorylation.

2 REACTIVE OXYGEN SPECIES AND FREE RADICALS

Free radicals are any species capable of independent existence and containing one or more unpaired electrons in the atomic or molecular orbitals. Oxygen molecule is a biradical already in its ground state: it has two unpaired electrons with opposite spins in the outer orbitals of the two oxygen atoms. Without reduction the oxygen molecule may also become excited through absorbing energy. The resulting singlet oxygen is not radical but diamagnetic.

In normal conditions, oxygenation reactions due to ground state bioxygen are rare: two electrons should be added at a time and that would assume a spin reversal of one of the two electrons. However, in enzymatic reactions one electron may be added at a time. Superoxide (O^{-2}) results from a one electron reduction, peroxide (H_2O_2; not a radical) from addition of two electrons, hydroxyl radical from addition of three electrons (and scission of the oxygen molecule) and water after addition of four electrons. The most reactive intermediate of the reaction chain is hydroxyl radical, superoxide is also a free radical but less reactive.[1,2]

Superoxide anions are produced constantly in various tissues as a result of both enzymatic and autooxidative processes. During the last years, special attention has been given to superoxide anion production under hypoxic states.[2]

H_2O_2 is generated in various enzymatic reactions.[1,2] It can be liberated also from reactions of various respiratory chains and from phagocytic cells. Superoxide anion and peroxide may also react in the presence of a transition metal catalyst to produce the hydroxyl radical species (the Fenton reaction).

Free radicals may also be centered around other atoms than oxygen.[3] They may be formed e.g. in various cytochrome P-450 catalyzed monooxygenation reactions. Reduced oxygen species and other inorganic and organic radicals are known to perturb cell functions due to their capability of changing the structure of macromolecules. Of the amino acids tryptophan, tyrosine, histidine and cysteine are sensitive to oxidative damage, of the fatty acids the polyunsaturated fatty acids. In nucleic acids oxidative damage may lead to structural changes which may result in mutations.

3 ANTIOXIDANTS AND OTHER FACTORS THAT PROTECT AGAINST OXIDATIVE DAMAGE

Adaptation to the use of various potentials of molecular oxygen in biochemical functions has evidently caused a need to adapt to the production of the reduced oxygen species. The actual biochemical part of this developed, so called antioxidant function is enzymatic, metabolizing harmful reactive oxygen compounds to less toxic form or repairing the damage caused by them. The rest is mostly nutrition dependent (vitamins E (including various tocols and tocotrienols) and C, beta-carotene and other carotenoids). Vitamin A is often included in this group of compounds. However, due to its hormone like tight homeostasis and low concentrations it can hardly be an essential antioxidant in tissues other than the liver. However, the role of vitamin A in cell differentiation and transformation is well known. Urate has also been shown to have antioxidant potential, however, it does not seem to be of chain-breaking nature.[4] Additionally, there are various sorts of chemicals which we receive with our food that may have antioxidant potential. These include e.g. various food additives.

There are three forms of superoxide dismutases in the eukaryotic cells: mitochondrial (containing manganese), cytoplasmic (containing zinc and copper) and extracellular (also containing zinc and copper). They convert two superoxide anions to molecular oxygen and hydrogen peroxide.[5,6] The extracellular form is assumed to be the most important antioxidant in the extracellular space e.g. in inflammatory conditions in which phagocytic cells have become activated to destroy microbes. The metal cofactors of the enzymes have essential roles in the reactions. The dismutation may also occur nonenzymatically. Glutathione peroxidase (selenoenzyme), some of the glutathione transferases and catalase metabolize organic and inorganic peroxides, the reaction products are an organic hydroxyl compound and water or water and molecular oxygen.[7,8] The relative activities of the various enzymes in different tissues and body fluids differ greatly. Carmagnol et al.[9] reported recently that the glutathione transferase dependent peroxidase activity was responsible for more than 80 per cent of the total peroxidase activity in the human liver, kidney cortex and skeletal muscle, in the kidney medulla for 57 per cent, in the adrenals for 22 per cent, in thrombocytes for 8.5 per cent. In a wide range of other tissues the transferase dependent peroxidase activity was non-measurable.

As many activities of the antioxidant enzymes are partially dependent on the availability of the metal cofactors, Se, Mn, Cu and Zn are often called antioxidant trace elements. They may also have enzyme independent roles in the antioxidant function.

What was said above, does not, necessarily, mean that no other enzymes are participating in the antioxidant activities: e.g. various aldehyde dehydrogenases detoxify toxic aldehydes which can result from lipid peroxidation. DNA damage caused by free radicals may be subject to repair by the DNA repair systems.

4 FACTORS AFFECTING THE LEVELS OF ANTIOXIDANTS IN TISSUES

Increased intake of selenium will lead to an increase in the activity of thrombocyte glutathione peroxidase in persons whose Se intake has been low.[10] In animal experiments it has been shown that several other enzyme activities are induced at the same time.[11] It has also been shown in laboratory animals that low Se intake leads to a compensatory increase in the glutathione transferase dependent peroxidase activity in such tissues where both the Se-dependent enzyme and the transferase are responsible for the peroxidase activity.[12] In tissues where the transferases do not show such an activity, Se deficiency cannot induce transferases with such an activity, either.[13]

Both hyperoxia and hypoxia are able to increase the activities of glutathione peroxidase, catalase and superoxide dismutase in blood. It is assumed that the basic mechanism behind this is related to the accumulation of reactive oxygen species in hyperoxic or hypoxic stress.[2]

Several genetic defects concerning the antioxidant enzymes are known. Mostly these enzymatic deficiencies are associated with granulomatous diseases resulting mainly from changed red cell and phagocytic cell functions.[14] The genetic and post-transcription regulation of the antioxidant enzymes are known rather well.[15-19] In Down's syndrome mutations related to the trisomy of chromosome 21 can result in an increase, decrease or no change in the activity of cytoplasmic superoxide dismutase.[20-22] It has been proposed that the changes in the enzyme activity might be related to the enhanced ageing process of the syndrome.

The fat soluble antioxidants are absorbed from the gut passively with the chylomicrons.[23] The transport of vitamin A from the liver is strictly regulated through the synthesis of retinol binding protein. Vitamin E is transported with lipoproteins to fat containing tissues and cell fractions. Beta-carotene is also associated with lipoproteins, its major storage site is the fat tissue.

Ascorbate is absorbed from the upper intestine through an active process. Its distribution is exceptional: although it is the most important chain-breaking antioxidant in serum, the highest concentrations are found in the adrenals, pituitary, corpus luteum, and retina where the concentrations are about 100 times higher than in serum. The absorption is dose dependent: of 200 mg/day approximately 150 mg are absorbed, of 3 g/day approximately 1200 mg. With an increase in the ascorbate uptake, the metabolic degradation is accelerated and the tubular reabsorption is reduced.[23]

Of the antioxidant trace elements Cu is absorbed mainly from the stomach.[24] The actively regulated step is the release of copper from the gastric cells to the blood stream. Approximately 50 % of the copper in the food is absorbed. The absorbed copper is transported to the liver as amino acid and albumin complexes. It leaves the liver bound to ceruloplasmin which has also some superoxide dismutase potential. The main excretory route for copper is through the bile. The highest copper concentrations are found in the liver, brain, kidney, heart and skeletal muscle. In Menkes' syndrome the absorption mechanism is perturbed, in Wilson's disease the secretion from the liver is disturbed due to the lack of ceruloplasmin synthesis.[25]

Manganese is absorbed through an active process in the upper intestine. Only a few per cent of the manganese in food is absorbed. In serum Mn is bound to transferrin. The highest Mn concentrations are in tissues containing plenty of mitochondria.[26] Mn is mainly excreted through the bile.

Zinc is also absorbed through an active process in the intestine. The type of food in the gut affects strongly the bioavailability of Zn. In the liver Zn is bound to metallothionein whose synthesis is in part regulated by Zn. Zn is secreted from the liver bound to metallothionein, amino acids or proteins. It is mainly excreted into the bile. In acrodermatitis enterohepatica, which is a complex illness and fatal without Zn treatment, the transport mechanism in the gut is deficient.[27]

The absorption of Se differs from those of the cationic elements described above. It is absorbed as an anion or as an organic complex. Its absorption is not under an active regulation. The absorbed selenate is quickly excreted through the kidneys. Selenium is bound to sulphur containing amino acids in food. These complexes are taken more readily than the inorganic compounds of selenium. Selenomethionine is also incorporated to the amino acid pool of the body. Due to that methionine bound selenium is excreted slowly from the body.[28] In serum Se is mainly transported bound to proteins. The highest tissue concentrations are found in the liver, kidney and spleen. Se is also methylated in the liver: the resulting trimethyl selenium ion is excreted through the kidneys. At higher uptake levels, the methylation capacity becomes saturated. As a consequence a volatile dimethyl metabolite is formed. It is excreted in the exhaled air. It has a particular garlic-type odor.[28]

5 ASSESSMENT OF THE ANTIOXIDANT FUNCTION

Measurement of all the major components of the antioxidant function is tedious even if all the related analytical problems were resolved. I have collected in Table 1 the major components that should be considered when planning to measure the antioxidant function in a comprehensive way.

The fact that measurement of all relevant factors at the same time is too demanding is a natural reason for the deep controversy in opinion on what roles free radicals in human morbidity actually have. A simpler technique would be to measure the antioxidant functions of tissue specimens in 'in vitro' conditions by adding a radical source directly to the specimen and following then the effects generated. Some trials in this direction have already been done.

To study the reactive species balance at any organ or tissue level would assume that the reactive compounds could be measured. In practice the techniques available are not, yet, suitable for clinical measurements in humans.

Additional problems arise from the biological and analytical problems of measurements of the various components of the antioxidant function. The analytical variation of measurement of vitamins and trace elements in serum or other specimens seems to be a manageable problem to day. Also reference materials and quality assurance schemes are becoming available. Measurement of separate fatty acids is laborious and such measurements may not easily become a part of large scale epidemiological studies.

Table 1 Measurement of Antioxidant Parameters

Vitamins	Enzymes	Other factors
* (A), E, C * Beta-carotene	* SOD, Catalase, GSHPOX, GSHT * Other detoxication and repair enzymes	* Se, Zn, Cu, Mn * GSH, -SH-groups * Urate, mannitol * Transferrin, ceruloplasmin * Other radical scavengers

Radical sources	Substrates for Reactions	Reaction Products
* Oxygen tension * Free radicals or other reactive species (direct or indirect)	* Separate fatty acids * Susceptible enzymes and nucleic acids	* Malondialdehyde * Diene conjugates (all or specific) * Fluorescing pigments * Exhaled pentane and ethane * Other LPO products * Inactivated enzymes * Adducted, altered or degraded nucleic acids

However, most of the other measurements (Table 1) are to-date nonstandardized. Lipid peroxidation is a complex phenomenon. Probably several of its intermediates and end-products should be measured at the same time. A classical example in this respect is the lipid peroxidation caused by CCl_4: 'in vitro' malondialdehyde is a main product. In 'in vivo' conditions, however, it cannot be found.[29] A probable explanation is that the reaction products differ in the two conditions. The analytical techniques used for malondialdehyde measurements do not, on most occasions, include a clean-up process to decrease the background absorption or fluorescence. No wonder that the reported 'normal' levels differ greatly.[30] Neither are the analytical techniques for the antioxidant enzymes standardized, yet.

The inter-individual variation is rather well known for antioxidant vitamins and trace elements. For the vitamins it seems to be quite remarkable.[31,32] For the lipid peroxidation and enzyme measurements this variation component is unknown.

For measurement of other tissue lesions than lipid peroxidation very few techniques are available to-date. With mass spectroscopy it has been possible to detect the binding of some carcinogenic compounds to tissue proteins.[33] In experimental conditions it has also been possible to measure the excretion in urine of such nucleic acid metabolites that indicate damage caused by inorganic or organic radicals.[33,34] These methods are, however, currently far from routine clinical tools.

6 CURRENT VIEWPOINTS

Most probably the analytical techniques we have for studies on health implications of reduced oxygen species and other reactive compounds will improve considerably in the near future. As discussed by Halliwell and Cutteridge,[35] there are, in principle, two options by which lipid peroxidation may be related to an illness or toxic exposure: the illness (or exposure) can cause enhanced lipid peroxidation due to an increase in cell degradation which in turn may lead to an increase in the amount of cell debris products which in part are lipid peroxidation products. Or the illness (or exposure) may enhance the rate of production of reduced oxygen species and other reactive compounds which then may result in enhanced lipid peroxidation and finally in cell death. Dormandy[36] (this volume) has further developed these concepts, suggesting that lipid peroxidation might in most conditions indicate normal cell catabolism.

On the other hand, it is very probable that there are conditions where reduced oxygen species or other reactive compounds in the body participate in the pathogenesis of various illnesses. As examples one may mention reperfusion injury in which the high redox potential developed during hypoxia leads to the acceleration of tissue damage at the phase of reperfusion.[35] Davies et al.[37] showed recently that thiobarbituric-acid-reactive material (malondialdehyde) was increased in acute myocardial infarction patients whose coronary artery could be made patent with streptokinase treatment, but decreased in patients whose coronary artery remained occluded. Another set of evidence comes from chemically induced cancer: a variety of exposures to organic chemicals are assumed to be carcinogenic due to the radical nature of the chemicals themselves or their metabolites in the body.[38] More recently it has been proposed that the oxidation of lipoprotein lipids in blood actually makes the low density lipoproteins susceptible to the uptake by the intima phagocytes which in turn may change to foam cells due to the accumulation of lipids in their cytosol.[39]

The research in this field is very active. But well planned extensive approaches are also needed to be more conclusive on the role of antioxidant function in human morbidity. There are several questions to be answered:

1. Can we prevent human illness by fortifying the antioxidant function through the means available (antioxidant vitamins and trace elements)? Probably the ongoing intervention studies will be more conclusive in this respect. 2. Are the physiological needs of everyone met when adequate food is available? This already seems to be more difficult to answer. The extremes seem to be those who consume much energy and those whose energy demands are low. 3. Are there needs to compensate for losses or decreased uptake of antioxidants caused by illnesses, medication or medical treatments or life-style (e.g. smoking or use of alcohol as the source of energy)? 4. Can we improve the natural history of illnesses by treating with antioxidants? All these four issues warrant scientific answers. The last one evidently will be very difficult to answer due to the complex etiology, diagnostics and ethical issues that are related to such studies on e.g. human cancer or atherosclerosis.

Finally, accepting that free radicals and other reactive species are factors involved in both physiological and pathophysiological processes, one must ask a pertinent question: Are we sure that we really can improve the antioxidant function for the whole organism's benefit? E.g. if intervening a cancer risk by treatment with antioxidants and succeeding in our intervention, does this also imply that the person will live longer or better? The most probable answer is that we do not know yet. Theoretically the (high) doses of the intervention to overcome the risks of one tissue may also lead to a disturbance in cell renewal in tissue with rapid turnover because of inhibited normal cell death. Evidently, we will learn more of these complex interactions when the results of the major intervention studies will become available.

7   REFERENCES

1.   W.A. Pryor, Annu.Rev.Physiol.,1986, **48**, 657.

2. H. Sies, ed., 'Oxidative Stress', Academic Press, London, 1985.
3. B. Halliwell, FASEB.J., 1987, 1, 358.
4. B. Frei, L. England and B.N. Ames, Proc.Natl.Acad. Sci.USA, 1989, 86, 6377.
5. S.L. Marklund, J.Clin.Invest., 1984, 74, 1398.
6. I. Fridovich, Adv.Enzymol., 1974, 41, 35.
7. B. Chance, H. Sies and A. Boveris, Physiol.Reviews, 1974, p. 527.
8. J.R. Prohaska, Biochim.Biophys.Acta, 1980, 611, 87.
9. F. Carmagnol, P.M. Sinet and H. Jerome, Biochim. Biophys.Acta, 1983, 759, 49.
10. O.A. Levander, G. Alfthan, H. Arvilommi, C.G. Gref J.K. Huttunen, M. Kataja, P. Koivistoinen and J. Pikkarainen, Am.J.Clin.Nutr., 1983, 37, 887.
11. A-S. Chung and M.D. Maines, Biochem.Pharmacol., 1981, 30, 3217.
12. A. Mehlert and A.T. Diplock, Biochem.J., 1985, 227, 823.
13. C.D. Thomson, S.M. Steven, A.M. van Rij, C.R. Wade and M.F. Robinson, Biochem.Int., 1988, 16, 83.
14. D.R. Raine, In: 'Chemical Diagnosis of Disease', S.S. Brown, F.L. Mitchell and D.S. Young, eds, Elsevier, Amsterdam, 1979, Chapter 18, p. 927.
15. R.B. Wadey and J.K. Cowell, Nucleic Acids Res., 1989, 17, 3332.
16. O.W. McBride, A. Mitchell, B.J. Lee, G. Mullenbach and D. Hatfield, Biofactors, 1988, 1, 285.
17. S.L. Marklund, L. Tibell, K. Hjalmarsson, G. Skogman, A. Engström and T. Edlund, Basic Life Sci., 1988, 49, 683.
18. J.K. Wen, T. Osumi, T. Hashimoto and M. Ogata, Physiol.Chem.Phys.Med.NMR, 1988, 20, 171.
19. C.G. Faulder, P.A. Hirrell, R. Hume and R.C. Strange, Biochem.J., 1987, 241, 221.
20. J.L. Huret, J.M. Delabar, F. Marlhens, A. Aurias, A. Nicole, M. Berthier, J. Tanzer and P.M. Sinet, Hum. Genet., 1987, 75, 251.
21. K. Miyazaki, T. Yamanaka and N. Ogasawara, Clin.Genet., 1987, 32, 383.
22. A.D. Ackerman, J.C. Fackler, C.M. Tuck-Muller, M.M. Tarpey, B.A. Freeman and M.C. Rogers, N.Engl.J.Med., 1988, 318, 1666.
23. L.J. Machlin, ed., 'Handbook of Vitamins', Marcel Dekker, New York, 1984.
24. G.T. Strickland, W.M. Bechner and M.L. Leu, Clin. Sci., 1972, 43, 617.
25. F.W. Sunderman, In: 'Chemical Diagnosis of Disease', S.S. Brown, F.L. Mitchell and D.S. Young, eds, Elsevier, Amsterdam, 1979, Chapter 19, p. 1009.
26. World Health Organization, 'International Programme on Chemical Safety, Environmental Health Criteria 17, Manganese', WHO, Geneva, 1981.
27. K.M. Hambidge, Phil.Trans.R.Soc.Lond., 1981, B294, 129.

28. World Health Organization, 'International Programme on Chemical Safety, Environmental Health Criteria 58, Selenium', WHO, Geneva, 1987.
29. R.O. Recknagel and A.K. Ghoshal, Lab.Invest., 1966, 15, 132.
30. C.R. Wade and A.M. van Rij, Clin.Chem., 1989, 35, 336.
31. W. Lee, K.A. Davis, R.L. Rettmer and R.F. Labbe, Am.J.Clin.Nutr., 1988, 49, 286.
32. N.V. Dimitrov, C. Meyer, D.E. Ullrey, W. Chenoweth, A. Michelakis, W. Malone, C. Boone and G. Fink, Am.J. Clin.Nutr., 1988, 48, 298.
33. H. Bartsch, K. Hemminki and I.K. O'Neill, eds, Lyon, IARC Scientific Publication, 1988, No. 89.
34. B.N. Ames, In: 'Medical, Biochemical and Chemical Aspects of Free Radicals', O. Hayaishi, E. Niki, M. Kondo and T. Yoshikawa, eds, Elsevier, Amsterdam, 1989, Vol. 2, p. 1453.
35. B. Halliwell and J.M.C. Cutteridge, Lancet, 1984, i, 1396.
36. T.L. Dormandy, Lancet, 1988, i, 1126.
37. S.W. Davies, K. Ranjadayalan, D.G. Wickens, T.L. Dormandy and A.D. Timmis, Lancet, 1990, 335, 741.
38. International Agency for Research on Cancer, 'IARC Monographs on the Evaluation of Carcinogenic Risks to Humans', Lyon, 1987, Supplement 7.
39. S. Ylä-Herttuala, W. Palinski, M.E. Rosenfeld, S. Parthasarathy, T.E. Carew, S. Butler, J.L. Witztum and D. Steinberg, J.Clin.Invest., 1989, 84, 1086.

Free Radicals, Lipid Peroxidation and Human Disease

T. L. Dormandy

DEPARTMENT OF CHEMICAL PATHOLOGY, WHITTINGTON HOSPITAL,
LONDON NW5 1RD, UK

1 RETROSPECT

Free radicals are a chemical species with an unpaired electron in their structure. For many years this meant that they were forbidden to exist. The obligatory pairing of electrons, closely related to the doctrines of valency and molecular weight, was part of the foundations of modern chemistry. Electrons can be conceived as poles of a magnet; and, however many times you break a magnet between its north and south pole, each of the two fragments will instantly reconstitute both poles. The same had to be true of electrons.

But, as happens in science, hardly had the law of electron pairing been enunciated when exceptions began to be noticed[1]. In particular, Michaelis, eponymous hero of enzyme kinetics, showed in the late 19-thirties that in some oxidation-reductions electron pairs were transferred from reductants to oxidants not as pairs but as unpaired electrons[2]. These were not free-radical reactions as we now understand the term since the separated electrons almost instantly reunited; but they nevertheless established that free radicals could exist.

The real break-through came in the early 19-forties when Farmer and his team[3], working in the laboratories of the British Rubber Producers Association, showed that rancidification, an age-old mystery, was a free-radical-mediated self-catalysing chain autoxidation. The discovery revolutionised industrial chemistry; but it took another quarter century before it began to make an impact on biology and medicine[4]. Even in the early 19-sixties a speculative article in The Lancet entitled "Biological rancidification" aroused a storm of protest.

I am recalling this not because of its slight anecdotal interest but because the reasons for looking at biological free radicals with scepticism are as valid today as they were twenty-five years ago. It has become fashionable in recent years to see free radicals everywhere, especially in diseases which cannot be explained in terms of more orthodox concepts. It is worth emphasizing therefore that free radicals are still an "improbable" biological species; that their generic role is different from other biochemical species; and that their methodology is still fraught with uncertainties.

2 IMPROBABILITY

Representations of free-radical sequences and of classical lipid peroxidation in particular can be misleading. They tend to show fast, sometimes explosively fast self-catalysing chain reactions in which hundreds, thousands, or millions of free radicals tumble over each other at great speed. This can and does happen, of course, once you have generated a few chain-initiating free radicals. But the diagrams do not always emphasize that very special conditions have to prevail for chain-initiation, the generation of a first free radical. This applies especially to organised biological material[5].

The main chemical ingredients of lipid autoxidation are, of course, all present in abundance in organized living cells. They contain a high proportion of highly unsaturated fatty acids; they are shot through with transitional metal complexes; and there is almost always a virtually limitless supply of oxygen. But the essence of biological organization is that the components of potentially dangerous interactions are kept strictly apart - *ie,* compartmentalised. The importance of this can easily be demonstrated with any fresh tissue. Left on the bench even at room temperature it may take days or weeks to go rancid. But simple homogenisation may trigger off the process within minutes.

But structural organization is not the only factor that makes free-radical generation improbable. Structures which are especially vulnerable - such as membranes - are amply provided with antioxidants and free-radical scavengers. And most importantly, in my opinion, no single reaction in normal intermediate metabolism generates a large enough single quantum of energy to sunder a stable electron pair. So how do potentially chain-initiating free radicals arise in a normal, organized, living cell? My own answer would be that in a normal, organized living cell they do not arise. Let me try to explain this seemingly heretical statement.

3 FREE RADICALS AND STRUCTURAL DAMAGE

That free radicals can cause severe and irreversible structural damage to cells, tissues and organs has been recognised for many years: indeed, it was the reason why biologists and doctors first took an interest in the species. But it is still not always appreciated that the relationship in reciprocal. In other words, not only do free radicals cause structural damage but also some degree of structural damage is probably essential for free-radical generation. There are two reasons for this.

First, for a free radical to be generated - and I am now talking of first, that is potentially chain-initiating free radicals - the chemical ingredients of free-radical generation must not only be present but must also be able to interact: in other words there must be some degree of "decompartmentalization". Second, some physico-chemical event must set free a sufficiently large single quantum of energy to separate a previously stable electron pair. I think that the only occasion when this happens in a structurally organized living cell is when there is some structural disruption.

Perhaps it is worth recalling in this connection that even though much remains to be learnt about the chemical reactions which lead to the assembly of an organized biological structure (*eg*, a cell), there is no doubt that the overall process is highly energy-consuming. Some of the energy expanded remains latent in the finished structure. Conversely, structural damage and disruption is always a highly exergonic event: it sets energy free and often in a large single quantum. We often picture cell death as a kind of passive falling apart. In reality organized biological structures do not fall apart. They explode. And molecular explosion may be necessary to initiate a free-radical reaction.

All this may conjure up a somewhat forbidding image of free radicals as the products or the agents of destruction; and this image is reinforced daily not only in the scientific and medical but also in the lay press. To some extent it is of course a legacy of industrial lipid chemistry, the parent science of free-radical biology and medicine. The main and indeed the only practical objective of Farmer and his colleagues in their pursuit of rancidification was to find ways of preventing it. In the industrial context lipid peroxidation is almost always a disaster, involving the irreversible loss of precious unsaturated oils and fats. But biochemists and doctors have done little to modify this image.

You can walk into any pharmacy and you will find on display rows of "tonics" and "rejuvenators" most of which claim to have antiperoxidant or free-radical-scavenging properties. In Britain house-keeping magazines overflow with advertisements for agents which will protect against free-radical damage. One may smile at all this in a superior manner; but in fact the sales talk echos (even if it also distorts) scientific literature. Lipid peroxidation is a "bad" thing because it damages or destroys tissues. Mechanisms which prevent lipid peroxidation are *ipso facto* described not as "inhibitory" but as "protective". Before even examining the evidence it is assumed in the general medical literature that disease is associated either with circumstances which promote peroxidation or with inadequate antioxidant (or antiperoxidant) "protection". Let me try - at the risk of spelling out the obvious - to correct this picture.

4 THE SURVIVAL VALUE OF CELL DESTRUCTION

The survival of complex organisms depends critically on the continuous renewal - that is on the continuous turnover - of its constituent units; and this continuous renewal depends entirely on continuous destruction. Theoretically, of course, one could picture an arrangement based on production: an organ, for example, could maintain a constant cell complement if every new cell produced led to the destruction of an old cell. It just so happens that this is not how nature operates - at least not in the human organism. In man normal cell turnover is determined by - and continually adjusted to - the rate of cell destruction. (The same is true of smaller units like subcellular particles whose turnover is generally considerably faster than that of cells.) I need hardly remind you that very little is known about the mechanisms responsible for maintaining this destruction-led equilibrium; but if one had to write a kind of "job description" on would come up with two essential requirements.

First a self-destruct mechanism would have to be built into every cell. This would have to be capable of being triggered into action not only by the expiry of the cell's normal life span but also by a wide range of abnormalities which might make the premature destruction of the cell desirable. Let me emphasize that it would be no good to have this mechanism confined to liver cells or red blood cells or any other specific kind of cell. Even nerve cells which are not apparently renewed after a certain age have an internal turnover of their subcellular structures. It would be essential for the self-destruct mechanism not to be activated during the cell's normal life span.

Second, the self-destruct mechanism would have to be capable of generating specific chemical products not generated in the course of normal cell metabolism. These would act as signals for the replacement of the cell destroyed.

All this may sound rather theoretical; and the fact that free-radical-mediated lipid peroxidation "fits the bill" does not of course mean that free-radial-mediated lipid peroxidation is the mechanism responsible. But I would suggest that if lipid peroxidation did not exist as a potential self-destruct mechanism which also generates a host of potential chemical messengers, then something similar would have to be invented[6].

There are of course a number of specific instances where lipid peroxidation is already known to be critically involved in this kind of programmed self-destruction. Phagocytes by polymorphonuclear leucocytes is one[7]; platelet aggregation is another[8]. And failure of the self-destruct process may be an important aetiological factor in many diseases. Let me briefly and in a rather simplistic way consider two.

5 FREE RADICALS AND CANCER

Cancer is a two-faced problem. First, a wide variety of "causes" are known which can initiate and promote the carcinogenic process at the cellular level. Second, there are clearly powerful protective mechanisms which are capable of destroying and eliminating cells which have undergone cancerous change. Clinical cancer can be due to active carcinogenesis so powerful that it overwhelms the normal eliminating process. But it can also be due to the failure of this process to overcome "normal" carcinogenic influences. I would suggest that carcinoma of the cervix, for example, is usually "caused" not by any particularly powerful carcinogenic agent but by a decline in the protective potential that is built into the normal cervical epithelium.

Inevitably perhaps cancer has always been one of the main targets of free-radical research; and I cannot review all the links which have been established between the disease and free-radical activity. But I would like to draw your attention to one development which is relevant to what I have suggested.

When lipid peroxidation in cancer was first studied it was confidently expected that cancer cells would be more active in generating free radicals than normal cells and more susceptible to free-radical damage. I can only describe the "reason" for this expectation as psychological, a form of mental conditioning. Cancer was recognised as a "destructive" process. Free radicals too were known as "destructive". The two would surely be positively linked. In a wide range of experimental systems - now even in human cancer - the relationship is the exact reverse. Cancerous cells in most types of cancer are much more resistant to lipid peroxidation than normal cells[9,10]: they are better "protected", to use an increasingly meaningless terminology. What the underlying mechanism is remains uncertain; but the fact is not in serious doubt. We have to envisage the possibility that many or most clinical cancers in man depend not on the carcinogenic transformation of cells (which may be extremely common and not in itself dangerous) but on the failure of these transformed cells to activate their built-in self-destruct mechanism. And if, as I believe, this self-destruct mechanism involves or even depends on free-radical-mediated lipid peroxidation then its potential survival value would be obvious. In this connection it is perhaps worth mentioning that quite empirically we may already be using this knowledge since both X-irradiation and the majority of pharmacological anticancer agents are powerful promoters of lipid peroxidation: in other words they may be performing (very crudely) what should be a built-in normal function of all cells.

This does not of course mean that lipid peroxidation is a "good thing" any more than X-irradiation in itself is a "good thing". But it does mean that lipid peroxidation is almost certainly a normal mechanism; and that it almost certainly plays an important part in the programmed destruction of abnormal and potentially dangerous as well as of time-expired cells. Conversely, diseases can be caused by bad programming in either direction - *ie*, both by excessive and by inadequate peroxidation.

6 FREE RADICALS AND AGEING

Before I summarise and try to peer into the future I should like to mention another field in which free-radical activity is often misinterpreted. Ageing is, of course, a notoriously treacherous subject; but it is also an important one. I should like to make it clear that I am not talking of life-span. Contrary to what is often implied, life-span and ageing are only incidentally related. The life-span of a species is encoded in its genes, and nothing short of genetic engineering can conceivably change it. But within this life-span there is a degenerative process which, for want of a better word, we can call ageing and which may be an important predisposing cause of many age-related diseases.

There is undoubtedly a link between ageing and free-radical activity in many animal species[11]; and a great deal of publicity has been given to the possibility that antioxidants and other types of free-radical scavengers might have an "anti-ageing" effect in man. I do not want to dismiss the possibility offhand; but I do want to make one point that is often overlooked.

Supposing we did find an agent which would suppress lipid peroxidation *in vivo* and delay ageing at the cellular level. This might be beneficial in diseases in which cell survival was abnormally shortened - *eg*, in certain hemolytic states. But the prolongation of cell survival beyond the normal would be or could be just as harmful to the organism as a whole as premature cell destruction. Prolonged cell survival would slow down cell turnover and could leave the individual with an old and inefficient cell population.

7 PROSPECT

Perusing current medical literature it is easy to feel exasperated with free radicals. They seem to be cropping up everywhere - in reperfusion injury, immune reactions, diabetes, atheroma, toxic states, rheumatoid arthritis and so on. And it has to be said that many of the findings reported and, even more, much of what is read into the findings is pretty meaningless. Almost every pathological process is associated with abnormalities of cell turnover, either an increase or a decrease or both. Inevitably, in my opinion, this means abnormal free-radical activity. In itself such a finding means very little. What we need to know is the significance of the abnormality either in the causation of the disease or at least in the causation of important symptoms. In order to achieve this we need two things.

First, we need a better understanding of what free-radical activity means: in particular we need to get away from the still prevalent "good" and "bad" concept. Free radicals in themselves are no more "good" or "bad" than enzymes. It is inappropriate free-radical activity we should be chasing and if possible treating.

Second, we need a much improved methodology. At present almost all free-radical research in biology and medicine is based on indirect evidence and some of it is pretty remote. Supposing one finds increased superoxide-dismutase activity in some disease. Does that indicate increased free-radical generation which can certainly induce increased enzyme activity? Or does it mean diminished free-radical activity since the enzyme is known to scavenge free radicals? There is no way of knowing: you can take your pick according to your preconceptions. Evidence of lipid peroxidation is still based almost entirely on the measurement of thiobarbituric-acid reactivity and total diene conjugation. Neither is specific enough for what should be the next targets in free-radical research.

So what is the answer? Eventually, one must hope, electron-spin-resonance spectroscopy (with or without spin trapping) will provide a methodology applicable to clinical material. At the moment it is still far too cumbersome and far too expensive. In the mean-time we need better and more specific free-radical markers. I should like to think that trace-element research may provide such markers as a "spin-off". Many trace elements - not only iron and copper but also selenium, aluminium, cadmium, manganese and perhaps others - play a critical role in free-radical generation in general and in lipid peroxidation in particular. It would be a great advance if we could establish more and stronger links.

8 REFERENCES

1. D.H.Hay and W.A. Waters, Chem. Rev., 1937, 21, 1692.
2. B.Chance, in 'Free Radicals in Biological Systems' ed. N.S. Blois), Academic Press, London, 1961.
3. C. Walling, in 'Free Radicals in Solutions', Wiley & Sons, New York, 1957.
4. T.L. Dormandy, J. Roy. Coll. Phys. Lond. 1989, 23, 221.
5. T.L. Dormandy, Lancet, 1978, i, 647.
6. T.L. Dormandy, Lancet, 1988, ii, 1126.
7. M.B. Babior, New Engl. J. Med. 1978, 298, 659.
8. A.W. Segal & T.J. Peters, Lancet, 1967, i, 1363.
9. T.F. Slater, F. Bajardi, C. Benedetto, G. Bussolati, S. Cianfano, M.U. Dianzani, B. Ghiringello, G. Nohammer, W. Rojanapo and E. Schauenstein, FEBS Lett., 1985, 187, 267.
10. K.H. Cheeseman, M. Collins, K. Proudfoot, T.F. Slater, G.W. Burton, A.C. Webb and K.U. Ingold, Biochem. J., 1986, 235, 507.
11. T.F. Slater, 'Free Radicals in Tissue Injury', Pion, London, 1972.

Metal–Proteoglycan Interactions in the Regulation of Renal Mesangial Cells: Implications for Metal-induced Nephropathy

Douglas M. Templeton

DEPARTMENT OF CLINICAL BIOCHEMISTRY, UNIVERSITY OF TORONTO, TORONTO, CANADA M5G 1L5

1 INTRODUCTION

As the catalogue of growth-regulating molecules expands, the potential targets of metal toxicity accordingly increase in number. Our earlier understanding of the toxic actions of metals has served well in elucidating some chemical principles underlying the basis of these adverse effects. These have been described in terms of ionic interactions with nucleic acids, poisoning of enzyme activities by thiol binding, or disruption of catalytic action by isomorphous replacement of other metal cofactors. This picture must now be revised to include potential effects on molecules of diverse function. Possible targets include peptide hormones and receptors, growth factors and transcriptional effectors (notably Zn finger proteins)[1], and other sites in signal transduction pathways (*eg* those homologous to the cytosolic domain of the epidermal growth factor receptor) and cell adhesion molecules (*eg* laminin and N-CAM) with Cys-rich domains.

In the present report, we consider the role of proteoglycans (PGs) as another important class of growth regulators in some, if not all cells. We advance the hypothesis that, by virtue of their highly anionic character, PGs are subject to modulation by charge reduction as a consequence of metal ion binding. In the renal glomerulus, several classes of PGs are produced to serve a variety of purposes, including contributions to the structure and function of the glomerular matrices and probable autocrine or paracrine control of mesangial cell growth. Therefore, we have investigated the effects of divalent metals on the biosynthesis, secretion and anti-mitogenic properties of PGs, using isolated glomeruli and cultured glomerular mesangial cells as models with toxicological implications. To underscore the implications for nephrotoxicity of PG charge reduction, we will first briefly describe the role of the mesangial cell in renal dysfunction, and the known effects of PGs on this cell.

Mesangial Cells in Toxic Nephropathy

Mesangial cells participate in the regulation of glomerular filtration by at least two mechanisms. The contractility of these smooth muscle-like cells facilitates regulation of capillary flows and filtration surface area[2]. They also elaborate a unique extracellular matrix, the mesangium, through which a significant portion of the forming plasma filtrate passes[3]. Loss of contractility is expected to impair the control of glomerular filtration rate, while abnormal matrix synthesis can lead to accumulation and sclerosis. This latter change is a characteristic of most if not all progressive renal disease, and has been described as a feature of the limited repertoire of response to injury mounted by the glomerulus[4]. Because the mesangial cell is quiescent in the healthy mammalian glomerulus[5], its activation is a common event in glomerular pathology. The consequent synthesis of matrix components, including PGs, if unchecked may progress to the obliteration of functional tissue. From this perspective, the growth suppressive factors maintaining mesangial cell quiescence are of paramount importance in understanding the mechanisms of renal disease. Prime candidates for such factors are the PGs themselves (vide infra), that are released from glomerular epithelial, mesangial and endothelial cells. Completing this picture, the mesangial cell may respond to the composition of the matrix itself[6], altering the expression of PGs in a manner determined in part by the cell's surroundings[7]. From this description it should be clear that the essential metabolic and regulatory activities of glomerular PGs are in a careful balance that may be tipped by interactions with toxic metals.

PG Structure and Mesangial Cell Function

PGs consist of one or more glycosaminoglycan chains on a protein core. In the glomerulus, glycosaminoglycans of the chondroitin, dermatan and heparan sulphate (HS) series are produced, giving rise to several distinct populations of PGs[6,8]. A constant background of carboxylate functionality on every second residue, with variable sulphation of both hexosamine and iduronic acid residues, imparts to all these glycosaminoglycans a significant negative charge and anionic polyelectrolyte behaviour. Polyelectrolyte properties dominate the solution chemistry of the PGs[9], and together with their net negative charge contribute to most if not all of the biological activities of these multifunctional molecules [10]. Obligatory counter-ion binding can reduce the net charge density of the glycosaminoglycan, and potentially interfere with biological functions.

Numerous reviews of PG function are available[10-12]. With respect to mesangial cell physiology, physicochemical properties of the PGs contribute to maintenance of the structural integrity of the mesangial matrix by means of binding interactions with Type IV collagen, laminin and fibronectin[13]. The counter-ion environment of the polymer establishes an osmotic gradient that affects the hydration properties of the matrix. The mesangial matrix also plays a significant role in plasma ultrafiltration, along with the glomerular basement membrane (GBM), and so the contribution of the PGs to electrostatic selectivity in filtration through the GBM[14] may be extended to include a similar role in the mesangium. PGs also exhibit growth-regulatory activity, although the mechanisms are known in less detail[10]. They are expressed on most cell surfaces, and may serve in cell recognition, adhesion and receptor capacities. Their behaviour may be a direct effect of interaction of soluble and (or) matrix PGs with cells, or an indirect effect of growth factor binding.

Medium conditioned by glomerular epithelial cells was shown to contain heparinase-sensitive inhibitors of mesangial cell growth[15], leading to speculation on a paracrine role for HS in maintaining mesangial cell quiescence. Of about 20 cell types tested, heparin showed a potent antiproliferative activity only in vascular smooth muscle cells and mesangial cells[16]. Recently HS from bovine lung has been shown to inhibit mesangial cell growth[17]. The mechanism(s) by which this effect is exerted remains to be elucidated. Evidence has been presented for receptor-mediated endocytosis of heparin by vascular smooth muscle cells[18]. A novel mechanism for internalization of HS by cultured hepatoma cells has been proposed[19], involving receptor binding of a myoinositol phosphate linked to the HSPG core protein. The appearance of HS in the nucleus correlated with inhibition of growth of log phase cells, and the block was in G_1 prior to the G_1/S boundary[20]. Heparin has been shown to delay entry of aortic smooth muscle cells into S phase, probably acting in late G_1, and to reduce the number of cells exiting G_o[21]. Inhibition by heparin of the proliferative response of these cells to phorbol esters, but not to epidermal growth factor, suggests that the PG inhibits a protein kinase C-dependent mechanism.

2 MATERIALS AND METHODS

Glomeruli were isolated from male Wistar rats by graded sieving as described[8]. Mesangial cell cultures were initiated essentially as described by Striker and Striker[22]. Glomeruli from younger rats (100 g) were cultured in RPMI 1640 medium in a humidified CO_2 atmosphere, containing 20% calf serum and antibiotics.

Mesangial cells were subcultured by trypsinization at 28 days, and for the experiments reported here were used before the tenth passage. Details are reported elsewhere[7].

PGs were labelled by addition of carrier-free [^{35}S]-sulphate to mesangial and glomerular cultures. Newly synthesized PGs were extracted, purified and identified by enzymatic and chemical degradation[8]. Protein and DNA synthesis were measured by the incorporation of [^{3}H]-leucine and [^{3}H]-thymidine, respectively, into trichloroacetic-precipitable material[23]. The preparation of metal stock solutions and their solubility under present culture conditions has been described[23]. To determine their effects on PG synthesis in isolated glomeruli, metal salts were added at or near the concentration causing a 50% reduction in total protein synthesis over 16 h, as reported previously[23].

To study growth regulation in mesangial cells, sparsely plated cultures in 12-well plates were starved for 72 h in RPMI 1640 medium containing 0.4% calf serum. At the end of this time most cells were in G_o/G_1. They were then stimulated by feeding with 20% calf serum in fresh medium, and DNA synthesis was measured by a 1 h pulse of [^{3}H]-thymidine (2.5 mCi/L, 0.37 μmol/L). Heparin (pig intestinal mucosa; Sigma) and (or) $NiCl_2$ were added when desired at the time of stimulation with 20% serum. To study thymidine uptake, mesangial cells grown on glass coverslips were growth-arrested and fed with 20% calf serum for 2 h, and then exposed to 10 mCi/L [^{3}H]-thymidine (1.5 μmol/L) for 5 min as described by Castellot Jr. et al.[15].

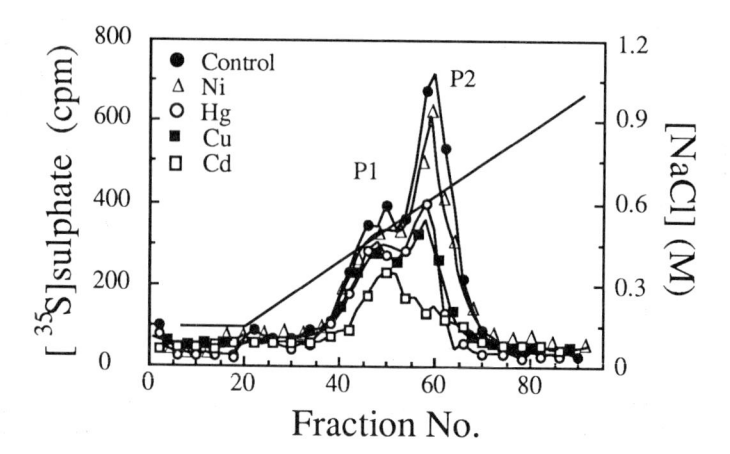

Figure 1 Effects of divalent metals on glomerular PGs

3 RESULTS AND DISCUSSION

PG synthesis by glomeruli

The effects on PG synthesis of Mn^{2+}, Co^{2+}, Ni^{2+}, Cu^{2+}, Zn^{2+}, Cd^{2+} and Hg^{2+} were investigated in the isolated rat glomerulus. Control glomeruli sulphated two populations of PGs, separable by ion exchange chromatography into those of higher and lower charge density (Fig. 1). The first peak is predominantly HSPG, whereas the second is mainly dermatan sulphate (DS)[8]. The different metals had differential effects on the two PG populations (Fig. 1). Whereas Mn, Co Ni and Zn had little or no effect on their relative proportions, Cu, Cd and Hg caused a more pronounced decrease in higher charge density DSPG. With Cd, the second peak was nearly completely eliminated. Because glomerular epithelial cells have been shown to produce mostly HSPG[24], while mesangial cells synthesize mostly DSPG, with lesser amounts of chondroitin sulphate and HSPG[7], these results may indicate preferential toxicity to the mesangial cells by the softer metals Cu, Hg and Cd. This possibility was evaluated in cultured mesangial cells.

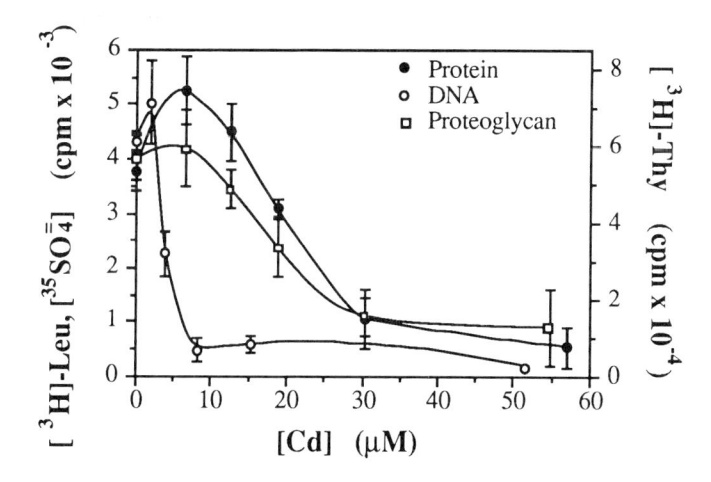

Figure 2 Effects of Cd on protein, proteoglycan and DNA synthesis

Effects of Cd on mesangial cells

Cadmium caused a 50% reduction in protein synthesis by mesangial cells over 16 h, at a concentration of about 25 µmol/L (Fig. 2). This is quite comparable to the corresponding value (30 µmol/L) in the intact glomerulus. Twenty µmol/L Cd^{2+} causes a 50% reduction in mesangial PG synthesis during this time, and at 30 µmol/L Cd^{2+}, synthesis is nearly obliterated. This is consistent with the loss of sulphation of higher charge density DS, of presumed mesangial cell origin, when the intact glomerulus is exposed to 30 µmol/L Cd^{2+}. DNA synthesis in these cells is particularly susceptible to Cd^{2+}, with an IC$_{50}$ of 5 µmol/L (Fig. 2). A comparison with the intact glomerulus was not possible, because in the freshly isolated glomerulus the cells remain in their quiescent *in vivo* state: incorporation of thymidine is minimal over the first several days[25].

These results lend support to the conclusion that toxicity to the mesangial cell underlies the Cd-induced decrease in DSPG synthesis by intact glomeruli. However, the decreased PG synthesis can be accounted for by a general decrease in protein and DNA synthesis by the cells, without the need to postulate specific targeting of PGs. In particular, there is no evidence that the mesangial PGs are qualitatively altered by the metal, and the post-translational events resulting in glycosaminoglycan chain synthesis appear to be intact. We have previously demonstrated that the sulphation of glomerular PGs *in vitro* is dependent on new synthesis of core protein, under conditions similar to those used here[8].

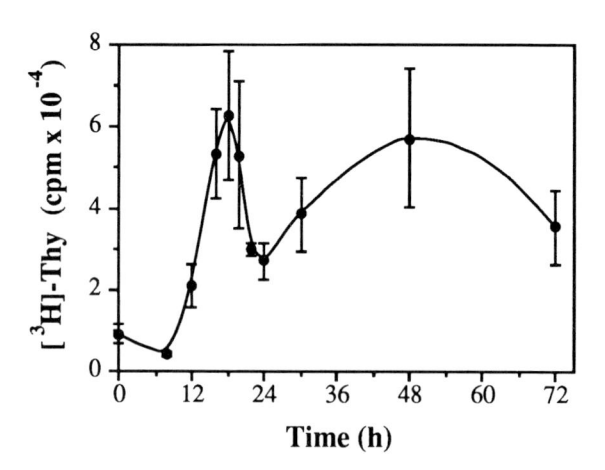

Figure 3 Recovery of DNA synthesis after serum-feeding of starved mesangial cells

Growth Suppression of Mesangial Cells by Heparin

Mesangial cells arrested in the G$_o$/G$_1$ phase of the cell cycle progress to S phase in approximately 18 h after feeding with serum, as indicated by a sharp increase in DNA synthesis at that time (Fig. 3).

Synchrony is reasonably well maintained for one complete cycle, as a second peak of DNA synthesis is clearly distinguishable approximately 30 h later. When heparin is added at the time of release, a dose-dependent suppression of the mitogenic response is seen (Fig. 4). Low concentrations of Ni have no significant effects on DNA synthesis in the stimulated cells. However, the presence of 30 µmol/L Ni^{2+} markedly blunts the suppressive effect of heparin (Fig. 4). In the absence of heparin, the stimulated mesangial cells take up ^{63}Ni. When 10 µmol/L heparin is present, the uptake is greatly reduced (Table 1).

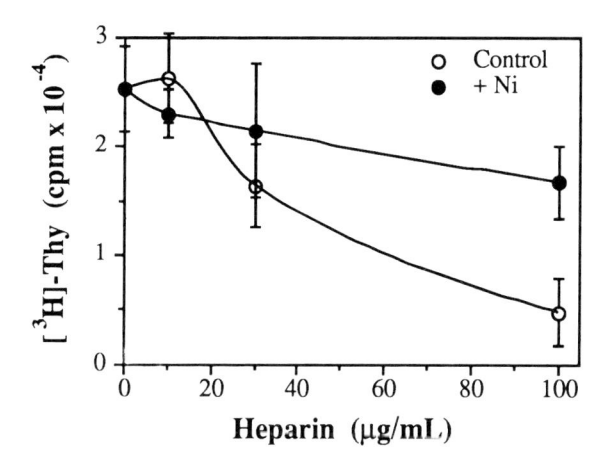

Figure 4 Effect of 30 µmol/L Ni on the suppression of mesangial cell growth by heparin.

Suppression of mesangial cells by medium conditioned by glomerular epithelia has been attributed in part to decreased thymidine transport, possibly in response to epithelial PGs[15]. In the present studies, the uptake of thymidine by stimulated mesangial cells was decreased by heparin, and again the effect was reduced by the presence of Ni^{2+} (Table 1). However, we have found the response of

Table 1 Interactions of heparin and Ni with respect to the uptake of Ni by confluent mesangial cells, and of thymidine by stimulated sub-confluent cells.

Label	[Heparin] (mg/L)	[NiCl$_2$] (mmol/L)	Uptake			Significance
^{63}Ni	0	10	31 ±	1	pmol	–
^{63}Ni	10	10	24 ±	3	pmol	p=0.001
[^{3}H]-Thy	0	0	5177 ±	632	cpm	–
[^{3}H]-Thy	10	0	3070 ±	742	cpm	p=0.02
[^{3}H]-Thy	0	10	3041 ±	737	cpm	p<0.02
[^{3}H]-Thy	10	10	3937 ±	765	cpm	n.s.

increased thymidine uptake to be less dramatic and less repeatable than the incorporation of the nucleotide into DNA.

Whether internalization is necessary for the growth regulating properties of heparin and HS is not known. Several mechanisms for extracellular actions must be considered. In particular, the binding of polypeptide mitogens by the heparin polyanion[26,27] is likely to contribute to the decreased mitogenic response in the stimulated cells. Any effect of heparin, whether due to growth factor binding, cell surface interaction, or internalization, is likely to be charge dependent[10] and therefore susceptible to metal ion binding. The prevention of cellular uptake of Ni by heparin, and the effects of the Ni-heparin system on thymidine transport, constitute indirect evidence for an extracellular action of heparin in the present study. We conclude that metal ion binding to extracellular PGs may result in enhanced stimulation of glomerular mesangial cells, with adverse consequences for renal function.

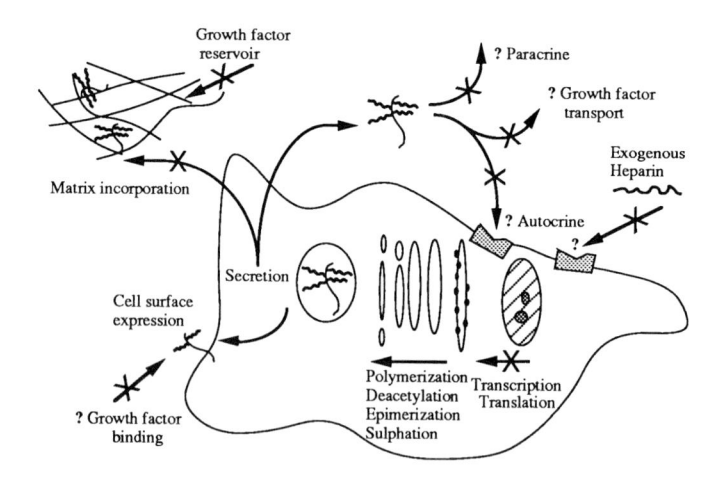

Figure 5 Possible sites of disturbed proteoglycan function after charge reduction by metal ions

4 SUMMARY

Metal ions are toxic to mesangial cells of the renal glomerulus. In part this toxicity is manifest by decreased production of PGs and interference with their diverse functions. Our present understanding of these events is summarized in Figure 5. Potential sites of interference are indicated by an 'X', and unproven functions or pathways are shown with a '?'. Inhibition of insertion of HSPG into GBM by Ni was demonstrated earlier, and interference with exogenous heparin is demonstrated here. Other interferences are presumptive, based on accessibility and the likely dependence of the function on charge density.

5 REFERENCES

1. F. W. Sunderman Jr. and A. M. Barber, Annals Clin. Lab. Sci., 1988, 18, 267.
2. J. I. Kreisberg, Mineral Electrolyte Metab., 1988, 14, 167.
3. P. Mené, M. S. Simonson and M. J. Dunn, Physiol.Rev., 1989, 69, 1347.
4. S. Klahr, G. Schreiner and I. Ichikawa, New Engl. J. Med., 1988, 318, 1657.
5. D. H. Lovett and R. B. Sterzel, Kidney Int., 1986, 30, 246.
6. E. Yaoita, Lab.Invest., 1989, 61, 410.
7. D. M. Templeton and A. Wang, Submitted, 1990,
8. D. Templeton and G. Castillo, Biochim. Biophys. Acta, 1990, 1033, 235.
9. D. Templeton, Can.J.Chem., 1987, 65, 2411.
10. E. Ruoslahti, J.Biol.Chem., 1989, 264, 13369.
11. A. R. Poole, Bichem.J., 1986, 236, 1.
12. E. Ruoslahti, Ann. Rev. Cell Biol., 1988, 4, 229.
13. R. Timpl, Eur.J.Biochem., 1989, 180, 487.
14. Y. S. Kanwar, Lab.Invest., 1984, 51, 7.
15. J. J. Castellot Jr., R. L. Hoover, P. A. Harper and M. J. Karnovsky, Am.J.Pathol., 1985, 120, 427.
16. J. J. Castellot Jr., D. L. Cochran and M. J. Karnovsky, J. Cell. Physiol., 1985, 124, 21.
17. G. C. Groggel, G. N. Marinides, P. Hovingh, E. Hammond and A. Linker, Am.J.Physiol., 1990, 258, F259.
18. J. J. Castellot Jr., K. Wong, B. Herman, R. L. Hoover, D. F. Albertini, T. C. Wright, B. L. Caleb and M. J. Karnovsky, J. Cell. Physiol., 1985, 124, 13.
19. M. Ishihara, N. S. Fedarko and H. E. Conrad, J.Biol.Chem., 1987, 262, 4708.
20. N. S. Fedarko, M. Ishihara and H. E. Conrad, J.Cell.Physiol., 1989, 139, 287.
21. J. J. Castellot Jr, L. A. Pukac, B. L. Caleb, T. C. Wright Jr and M. J. Karnovsky, J.Cell.Biol., 1989, 109, 3147.
22. G. E. Striker and L. J. Striker, Lab.Invest., 1985, 53, 122.
23. D. Templeton and N. Chaitu, Toxicology, 1990, 61, 119.
24. G. E. Striker, P. D. Killen and F. M. Farin, Transplantation Proc., 1980, 12 Suppl1, 88.
25. J. O. R. Nürgaard, Lab.Invest., 1987, 57, 277.

26 S. N. Mueller, K. A. Thomas, J. Di Salvo and E. M. Levine, *J.Cell.Physiol.*, 1989, **140**, 439.
27 R. Flaumenhaft, D. Moscatelli, O. Saksela and D. B. Rifkin, *J.Cell.Physiol.*, 1989, **140**, 75.

Application of an Organ Culture Matrix System to Neurotoxicity Studies in the Foetal Rabbit Midbrain

C. D. Hewitt, M. M. Herman, J. Savory, and M. R. Wills

DEPTS. OF PATHOLOGY, INTERNAL MEDICINE & BIOCHEMISTRY, UNIVERSITY OF VIRGINIA HEALTH SCIENCES CENTER, CHARLOTTESVILLE, VIRGINIA 22908, USA

1 INTRODUCTION

The *in vitro* culture of animal cells, tissues and organs is now a widely applied technique in many different disciplines, ranging from the basic sciences of cell and molecular biology to biotechnology. The field of toxicology, or more specifically neurotoxicology, is no exception, and many researchers are turning from the study of traditional *in vivo* animal model systems, which may be very expensive, to less expensive and perhaps more versatile *in vitro* culture systems.

The aim of the three dimensional organ culture system is to preserve the patterns of cell organisation and differentiation found *in vivo*, so that the explanted tissue closely resembles the parent tissue.[1] Proliferation and outgrowth of fibroblasts from the edge of the explant is discouraged by carefully selected culture conditions. The method of organ culture was originally designed for the investigation of embryonic organs and immature neonatal tissues by Fell et al[2] and was later extended to the study of normal mature or neoplastic tissues.[1,3-6] In this method, explants are cultured in a moist gas or air phase on the surface of a relatively large volume of stationary medium. In the presence of a large medium-gas interface, the rate of oxygen diffusion into the tissues is increased, and under these conditions cellular migration from the explant is considerably inhibited.

The "grid" technique was first introduced by Trowell in 1954.[3] The first grids were made of tantalum wire gauze; these were later replaced by the more rigid expanded metal grids comprised of stainless steel[7] or tantalum.[8] Skeletal tissues could be cultured directly on the grid, but softer tissues such as glands or skin were first explanted on strips of lens paper and then deposited on the grids. Lastly, the grids with their explants were placed in a culture chamber which was filled with medium up to the level of the grid.

The system used in the present study consisted of a porous foam matrix on a tantalum wire mesh platform, suspended over the central well of an organ culture dish. The nutrient medium bathed the foam matrix while circulating below the platform in the well of the culture dish and being retained by capillary action in the pores of the foam. This system favours cell growth and migration in three directions, and in the case of neoplasms, the matrix invasion by the explant may mimic the invasive characteristics of tumours *in vivo*.[1] However, neuronal foetal tissue, used in this study, migrates only superficially into the foam matrix, while astrocytes and fibroblasts may infiltrate more deeply.

The culture system has some advantages over those of monolayer and tissue culture namely individual explants can be subdivided and processed by multiple techniques, and can be chemically fixed and paraffin- or epoxy-embedded while still attached to their supporting matrices. Embedded tissue can then be sectioned on a microtome and studied with a variety of routine histological stains as well as by immunohistochemistry and electron microscopy.

2 MATERIALS AND METHODS

Medium

In the present study, explants were maintained in a 1:1 mixture of Dulbecco's Modified Eagle Medium (DMEM) and Ham's F-10 nutrient salts (both low glucose) (GIBCO Laboratories, Grand Island, NY), both reconstituted from powder and supplemented with 5 g/L D-glucose (Sigma Chemical Co., St. Louis, MO), 28 mmol/L sodium bicarbonate (GIBCO), 0.09 U/mL insulin (Sigma), 10 mmol/L N-2-hydroxyethyl-piperazine-N'-2-ethanesulfonic acid (HEPES)(Sigma), and young adult rabbit serum (10% v/v). This medium will be referred to as nutrient medium in the following text.

Reagents

Stock solutions of 25 mmol/L aluminium maltol[9] and 75 mmol/L maltol were prepared in deionized water and stored at 4°C. Working solutions of 440, 520 and 600 µmol/L Al maltol and 1.56 and 1.80 mmol/L maltol were filter-sterilized through a 0.22 µm filter (Nalgene Filterware, Nalge Co., Rochester, NY) and stored at 4°C for up to 10 days before use.

Tissue

New Zealand White rabbit foetuses were removed aseptically by Caesarian section at 24 days' gestation and placed in a 1:1 mixture of DMEM-F10 salts (no HEPES or insulin) at room temperature. Foetuses were rinsed in 70% ethanol and the crown-rump length was measured to confirm the gestational age.[10] Using medium size, straight scissors and forceps to remove the scalp, and fine scissors, watchmaker's forceps and curved microforceps to remove the skull and detach the brain, whole foetal brains were removed from the cranium and placed in supplemented medium, DMEM-F10 + 10% foetal calf serum (foetal calf serum, HyClone Laboratories Inc., Logan, UT). Under the dissecting microscope, coronal sections of the brain were taken at the level of the aqueduct. Explant cores of subaqueductal midbrain containing the oculomotor nucleus were removed from the coronal sections using a bone biopsy needle (Jamshidi needle, Pharmaseal Co., Glendale, CA) and placed in nutrient medium (10% RS). Explant cores were rinsed in DMEM-F10 salts + 50 mg/mL gentamicin for 5 min. and transferred to fresh nutrient medium. The final explants, 1-2 mm^3 sections of midbrain tissue, were placed on 5 mm^3 of Gelfoam (Upjohn, Kalamazoo, MI) set up on tantalum wire mesh platforms suspended over the central well of an organ culture dish (Organ Tissue Culture Dish, # 3037, Falcon, div. Becton, Dickinson and Co. Cockeysville, MD). The central well of the dish was filled with 2-mL of nutrient medium to just above the level of the platform so that the Gelfoam remained fully hydrated by capillary action. Approximately 3-mL of 1 X Hank's balanced salt solution (BSS) (GIBCO) were pipetted into the outer well.

After explanting, the organ culture dishes were placed in CO_2 water-jacketed incubators (Model # 3157, Forma Scientific, Marietta, OH or Model # 3321 NAPCO, Portland, OR) at 3.5-4.0% CO_2, 35.5-36.0°C and with a high relative humidity. Explants were left to attach to foams for 4 days before the initial exchange of spent medium. Thereafter, the spent medium was withdrawn and replaced with fresh medium three times per week. The Hank's BSS was replenished in the outer well of the culture dish in order to maintain the internal humidity.

Treatment

All foetal cultures were maintained *in vitro* for 15 days before treatment was commenced. Al-treated cultures were treated with a final concentration of either 11, 13 or 15 µmol/L Al maltol (50 µL of a working solution of Al maltol added to the central well of the culture dish containing 2-mL of medium). Maltol-treated cultures were treated with a final concentration of 39 or 45 µmol/L maltol (molar equivalent to 13 and 15 µmol/L Al maltol).

Treated cultures received Al maltol or maltol for 24 or 25 days, and were maintained for a total of 39 or 40 days *in-vitro* (established for 15 days plus 24 or 25 days' treatment). Control cultures were maintained on nutrient medium alone for the same period of time. A group of Al maltol- and maltol-treated cultures were carried for a further 10 days on nutrient medium alone (total of 50 days *in-vitro*) i.e., without the addition of Al maltol or maltol. Expected levels of aluminium in the fresh and spent nutrient medium were periodically confirmed by atomic absorption spectroscopy; details of this assay are reported elsewhere.[11]

Viable cultures were maintained for up to 50 days. Cultures were not carried for longer periods of time because neurotoxic effects were observed within this schedule. Healthy cultures remained translucent throughout the experiment, whereas the infrequent necrotic cultures invariably became opaque.

Fixation and Processing

Neuronal cultures, still attached to the foam matrix, were rinsed in Hank's 1 X BSS and sectioned prior to fixation. Approximately one third of each explant was processed for light microscopy, immunohistochemistry and electron microscopy.

Light Microscopy. A piece of each explant was fixed in 10% phosphate-buffered formalin for routine processing. Tissue was fixed at room temperature for 5 days, embedded in paraffin wax, mounted and 5 μm sections stained using either hematoxylin and eosin (H&E) or the Bielschowsky silver impregnation method for axons adapted for paraffin.

Immunohistochemistry. Tissue for immunohistochemistry was fixed in Bouin's fixative at room temperature for 24 hours and then transferred to 70% ethanol. Fixed tissue was processed within 2 to 3 days. A single 5 μm section was stained using H&E; consecutive unstained, 5 μm sections were immunostained according to the peroxidase-antiperoxidase method of Sternberger et al.[12] using a group of mouse monoclonal antibodies (Mabs). The panel of Mabs included 3 Mabs that recognize epitopes of neurofilament protein (NF-H/M) [SMI 31 recognizing phosphorylated (P+) epitopes; SMI 32, the non-phosphorylated, phosphorylation-dependent (P-) epitopes; and SMI 33, the phosphorylation-independent (Pind) epitopes]; 2 Mabs recognizing microtubule-associated proteins (tau and MAP2); and 2 anti-ß-tubulin Mabs, one recognizing the neuronal-associated class III isotype[13], and the other all mammalian ß-tubulin isotypes. Further details of the immunohistochemistry methods are reported elsewhere.[14,16]

Electron Microscopy. Tissue for electron microscopy was fixed at 37°C in a mixture of freshly prepared phosphate-buffered 2.5% glutaraldehyde and 1% paraformaldehyde (pH 7.2) which was allowed to cool gradually to room temperature; after 2 hours the tissue was transferred to sodium phosphate buffer and stored at 4°C. Following plastic embedding in epoxy resin (Epon 812), 1 μm semi-thin sections were obtained and blocks selected for ultrathin sections. The latter were stained on the copper grids with uranyl acetate and lead citrate and examined in a JEOL 100 S electron microscope.

3 RESULTS

Light Microscopy

Argyrophilic neuritic swellings and neuronal perikaryal inclusions were produced at 11, 13 and 15 μmol/L Al maltol. In maltol-treated and control cultures, perikaryal inclusions were absent and neuritic swellings were inconspicuous or absent. Treated cultures, carried for an additional 10 days without Al maltol, retained their neuronal perikaryal inclusions and neuritic pathology. We observed increased gliosis in cultures treated with 15 μmol/L Al maltol when compared with those receiving either 11 or 13 μmol/L Al maltol. As a result of this observation, the maximum concentration of Al maltol used was 15 μmol/L. At this concentration treatment could be continued for 25 days and viability was maintained.

Quantitation. The number of tangles produced in cultures treated with 11, 13 and 15 μmol/L Al maltol were counted by two observers and compared to untreated control cultures. Neurons were counted on one H&E section and silver positive tangles were tabulated on the next two serial sections, stained using the Bielschowsky silver method.

The percentage of neurons containing tangles in cultures treated with 11, 13 and 15 μmol/L Al maltol was 3, 7 and 7% of neurons respectively. The percentage of involved cells was found to be highly significant ($p<0.0001$, chi-square test) at all three levels of Al maltol when compared with control cultures.

Immunohistochemistry

Neuritic swellings and occasional perikaryal tangles were immunoreactive with Mabs against phosphorylated (P+), nonphosphorylated, phosphorylation dependent (P-) and phosphorylation independent (Pind) epitopes of the high (-H) and middle (-M) molecular weight neurofilament subunits (NF-H/M). By contrast these lesions were negative for microtubulin-associated proteins (tau and

MAP2) and ß-tubulin. These immunohistochemical findings are in agreement with previous immunohistochemical data from studies on Al maltol-treated rabbits, in which the compound was administered either intravenously[16] or intraventricularly.[15]

Electron Microscopy

Focal accumulations of bundles of straight 10 nm filaments were observed in occasional neuronal somata and neurites of aluminium treated explants. Aggregates of such intermediate filaments were not found in the maltol-treated or untreated explants.

4 DISCUSSION

Using the three dimensional organ culture system to maintain foetal rabbit midbrain explants we are able to analyse the same culture with multiple techniques, i.e. light microscopy, immunohistochemistry and electron microscopy.

In comparing our results with those of others, several authors have described the neurotoxic effects of aluminium in *in-vitro* models using organotypic cultures of foetal rabbit dorsal root ganglia[17] or dissociated tissue culture preparations of rat cerebrum[18] and mouse neuroblastoma cell lines.[19-21] Langui et al.[18] cultured rat brain neurons on astroglial feeder layers obtained by a lengthy two-step procedure. To the best of our knowledge, our group has been the first to apply the matrix culture system to studies of aluminium neurotoxicity. In this system, midbrain neurons and their associated astrocytes can be cultured for up to 50 days without overgrowth by astrocytes of the more fastidious neuronal elements.

In a review of the literature for purposes of comparing dosage levels of Al which have been applied *in vitro*, we have noted that Langui et al.[18] induced neurofibrillary tangles in 5 % of rat brain neurons with 0.01% aluminium chloride (750 µmol/L Al) in the medium after 14 days of treatment. These tangles showed reactivity towards Mabs recognizing each of the neurofilament subunits (NF-H, -M and -L) and were negative with anti-paired helical filament serum. Miller et al.[19] employed a neoplastic neuronal system, namely a mouse neuroblastoma cell line, which was capable of morphologic and biochemical differentiation in monolayer culture; they exposed these cells to medium containing aluminium phosphate at levels of 0.5-16 mmol/L Al.

Shea et al.[21] exposed murine NB2a/dl neuroblastoma cells, plated in chamber slides, to Al chloride and Al lactate at levels of 0.1-1.0 mmol/L. Separate cultures were examined by the Bielschowsky silver method, immunohistochemistry and electron microscopy. Silver stains demonstrated argyrophilic accumulations in the perikarya of many differentiated and undifferentiated cells. In two of these studies,[19,21] aluminium treatment resulted in the accumulation of straight intermediate (10 nm) filaments in the neuronal perikarya.

In order to perform these studies, the above authors were required to use a variety of culture systems.[18,19] For light microscopy, the cells were grown as a monolayer on individual sterile glass coverslips contained in glass Petri dishes. Electron microscopy was performed on cell monolayers grown on carbon-coated coverslips,[19] while growth rates were determined on cells cultured in plastic flasks. Saturated population densities (9 x 10^5 cells) were obtained rapidly, only 5 days after plating the cells at a density of 2 x 10^5.

Due to the nature of the monolayer culture system (both in the case of normal neurons cultured on astroglial layers and neuroblasts plated directly onto coverslips), the seeded cells multiplied rapidly and reached steady state within a week after plating. This factor alone limited the length of time the cells could be maintained *in vitro*, and thus shortened the length of time during which they could be treated. Therefore, in order to induce neurotoxic changes, higher concentrations (nonphysiological) of neurotoxins (0.1-16 mmol/L) were administered for a short period of time (<14 days). In contrast, using the three dimensional matrix system employed in the present study, cultures could be treated for at least 25 days with much lower concentrations of neurotoxins (11-15 μmol/L Al); i.e., at levels which are 10-100 times lower than those cited above.

Although we have only applied this matrix system to the evaluation of Al maltol-induced neurocytoskeletal changes in foetal rabbit midbrain culture, it could be easily adapted to the study of other neurotoxins. The availability of an *in vitro* system in which tangles can be consistently induced using aluminium should provide another approach for the study of the mechanism of aluminium neurotoxicity.

5 ACKNOWLEDGMENTS

Supported by Grant ES04464 of the National Institute of Environmental Health Sciences.

6 REFERENCES

1. L. J. Rubinstein, M. M. Herman and V. L. Foley, Am. J. Pathol, 1973, 71, 61.

2. H. B. Fell, P. N. Martinovitch and P. J. Gaillard, Methods Med. Res., 1951, 4, 233.
3. O. A. Trowell, Exp. Cell Res., 1954, 6, 246. 4. M-R. Roller, S. P. Owen and C. Heidelberger, Cancer Res., 1966, 26, 626.
5. F. L. Archer, Arch. Pathol., 1968, 85, 62.
6. M. Kalus and R. M. O'Neal, Arch. Pathol., 1968, 86, 52.
7. O. A. Trowell, Exp. Cell Res., 1959, 16, 118.
8. O. A. Trowell, Coll. Intern. CNRS, 1961, 101, 237.
9. M. M. Finnegan, S. J. Rettig and C. Orvig, J. Am. Chem. Soc., 1986, 108, 5033.
10. K. W. Hagen. "The Biology of the Laboratory Rabbit," Academic Press, 1974 New York and London, 1974, Chapter , p. 27.
11. C. D. Hewitt, K. Winborne, D. Margrey, J. R. P. Nicholson, M. G. Savory, J. Savory and M. R. Wills, Clin. Chem., in press.
12. L. A. Sternberger, P. H. Hardy, Jr., J. J. Cuculis & H. G. Meyer, J. Histochem. Cytochem., 1970, 18, 315.
13. A. Frankfurter, L. I. Binder & L. I. Rebhun, J. Cell Biol., 1986, 103, 273a (abstract)
14. D. V. Caccamo, M. M. Herman, A. Frankfurter, C. D. Katsetos, V. P. Collins and L. J. Rubinstein, Am. J. Pathol., 1989, 135, 801.
15. C. D. Katsetos, J. Savory, M. M. Herman, R. M. Carpenter, A. Frankfurter, C. D. Hewitt & M. R. Wills, Neuropathol. Appl. Neurobiol., 1990, in press.
16. R. L. Bertholf, M. M. Herman, J. Savory, R. M. Carpenter, B. C. Sturgill, C. D. Katsetos, S. R. VandenBerg & M. R. Wills, Toxicol. Appl. Pharmacol., 1989, 98, 58.
17. F. J. Seil, P. W. Lampert & I. Klatzo, J. Neuropathol. Exp. Neurol., 1969, 28, 74.
18. D. Langui, B. H. Anderton, J-P. Brion & J. Ulrich, Brain Res., 1988, 438, 67.
19. C. A. Miller & E. M. Levine, J. Neurochem., 1974, 22, 751.
20. G. M. Cole, K. Wu & P. S. Timiras, Int. J. Dev. Neurosci., 1985, 8, 23.
21. T. B. Shea, J. F. Clarke, T. R. Wheelock, P. A. Paskevich & R. A. Nixon, Brain Res., 1989, 492, 53.

Effects of Aluminium Maltol on Brain Tissue *in Vivo* and *in Vitro*

M. R. Wills, C. D. Hewitt, J. Savory, and M. M. Herman

DEPTS. OF PATHOLOGY, INTERNAL MEDICINE & BIOCHEMISTRY, UNIVERSITY OF VIRGINIA HEALTH SCIENCES CENTER, CHARLOTTESVILLE, VIRGINIA 22908, USA

1 INTRODUCTION

Aluminium is the most abundant metal and the third most common element in the earth's crust. The metal is normally present in vegetables, animal tissue and in untreated water. In some domestic tap-water supplies aluminium is present in high concentrations either naturally or, more commonly, because it has been added during the water purification (treatment) process as a flocculant. In addition to water, the major dietary sources of aluminium are from foods to which it has either been added or which naturally have a high content. The average daily intake of aluminium has been estimated to be approximately 9 mg per day in teenage and adult females and 12 to 14 mg per day in teenage and adult males.[1]

Absorption from the gastrointestinal tract is the main portal of entry into the body for this metal ion in normal subjects. The magnitude and importance of the uptake of aluminium from the nasal mucosa and lungs following the inhalation of dust is not, at this time, well defined. Particle size and the chemical state of aluminium would appear to be potentially important factors in both nasal and pulmonary uptake. The gastrointestinal tract is normally a relatively impermeable barrier to aluminium which has a very low fractional absorption rate in normal human subjects. The species of aluminium in the gastrointestinal tract appears to be a critical factor in the absorption process. The concomitant dietary intake of citrate appears to enhance the rate of absorption of aluminium from the gastrointestinal tract by an effect on species; specifically the formation of a chelate complex.

In the past decade attention has been drawn to aluminium because it is one of the potentially toxic acid-soluble metals that is leached from soil and rock by acid rain. High soil concentrations of aluminium potentially cause tree die-back injury by disturbing the soil nutrient cycle or by competing with calcium for binding sites on fine roots.[2] On aquatic life the lethal effects of acid rain appear to be due not only to acidity but also to the aluminium and other toxic metals that are mobilized at low pH from the soil and rock in the watershed area.[3] The toxicity of aluminium to fish depends primarily on its concentration and the simultaneous pH of their aquatic environment, with other factors playing contributory roles.[4-6] The critical factor is the pH of the aqueous environment which determines the speciation of aluminium.[7] Ionic aluminium, at a low pH, is the most toxic species to fish.[4] There is evidence, however, that a high concomitant calcium concentration appears to exert a protective action from the toxic effects of aluminium on both trees and fish.[2,8,9] Similarly, an excess of silicon over aluminium and the formation of hydroxy-aluminosilicate at pH 5 reduces the bioavailability and toxicity of aluminium.[10] A consideration of these observations on flora and fauna are of relevance to any consideration of the potential or known toxic effects of aluminium on the health of the human species.

During the past thirteen years it has been established that aluminium accumulates in the body tissues of some patients with chronic renal failure.[11,12] The tissue accumulation of aluminium in these patients is associated with the development of characteristic phenomena. The latter include a specific form of dementia, bone disease and an anaemia.[11-12] A higher prevalence of these phenomena occurred in those patients whose domestic water supplies contained significantly more aluminium and manganese with significantly less calcium and fluorine when compared with those patients who did not develop these disturbances.[13] A high soil and drinking water content of aluminium in combination with low contents of calcium and magnesium were also implicated as environmental factors in the etiology of two specific neurological disorders in three geographical locations in the western Pacific.[14] In these locations there was a high incidence of amyotrophic lateral sclerosis and parkinsonism in association with severe dementia. Aluminium has also been proposed as a potential toxin in the pathogenesis of Alzheimer's disease.[15-18] The potential existence of a link between Alzheimer's disease and aluminium has been recently highlighted by the report of a geographical relation between the prevalence of the disease and the aluminium concentration of drinking water.[19] It has also been reported that the mortality from motoneuron disease varies with the local water concentration of aluminium, especially among women.[20] An increase in the incidence of age-specific mortality from motoneuron disease, particularly among the elderly, has been reported in a demographic study.[21] The increase was attributed to environmental etiological factors and aluminium was one of the factors that was proposed to be of significance.

Abnormal processing of neuronal cytoskeletal proteins may be central to the pathogenesis of a wide spectrum of naturally occurring human neurodegenerations, including senile dementia of the Alzheimer's type (SDAT),[22-25] Parkinson's disease[26] and motoneuron disease (amyotrophic lateral sclerosis-ALS).[27-29] Aluminium-induced neurofibrillary degeneration bears some resemblance to human amyotrophic lateral sclerosis (ALS).[30,31] It has been proposed that the abnormal neurofilament phosphorylation of the lower motoneuron in ALS may be associated with an impairment of neurofilament transport in proximal axons, similar to the lesions of aluminium-induced neurofibrillary degeneration. In a recent study, there was some evidence that motoneuron pathology may be induced in cynomolgus monkeys after long-term maintenance on a low-calcium, high aluminium diet.[32] In our studies, we have investigated the changes in brain tissue following the accumulation of aluminium *in vivo* and exposure to aluminium *in vitro*.

2 EXPERIMENTAL STUDIES

In-vivo Studies

Long-term intravenous effect of aluminium maltol. We have studied the effects on central nervous system tissues of aluminium accumulation following its long-term intravenous administration in an animal (rabbit) model.[33] The administration of aluminium by the direct intravenous route was considered to be physiological in that it only "by-passed" the intestinal mucosal/serosal transport step which follows oral intake. The use of the intravenous route also allowed strict control of the amount of exposure to aluminium. The rabbit was chosen as the experimental animal because it was known to show neuropathological changes following the direct injection of aluminium into the central nervous system. Aluminium was given as a neutral water soluble complex (aluminium maltol). Irrespective of their weight, the rabbits (New Zealand Whites - all males) were given 3 mL of aluminium maltol solution intravenously three times a week (0.075 mmol/L of aluminium per injection) to give a total weekly load of 0.225 mmol/L aluminium (equivalent to 6.075 mg aluminium); another group of rabbits was given an equimolar dose of maltol. Tissues from an untreated control group of 15 age and sex-matched rabbits was used to obtain, for comparative purposes, brain tissue for microscopic examination and quantitative aluminium measurements. The treated rabbits were divided into two groups: aluminium maltol (AM)- and maltol (M)-treated. There were 22 rabbits in the AM-treated group and 17 in the M-treated group; they were maintained on intravenous injections for varying periods up to a maximum of 36 weeks. Small but significant increases in aluminium content of the hippocampus and brainstem were found in the AM-treated rabbits when compared with the untreated controls. A significant finding was the presence of prominent perikaryal argyrophilic masses (neurofibrillary tangles, NFT) in the neurons of the oculomotor nucleus (third cranial nerve nucleus, OMN) at the mesencephalic level in 3 of 10 of the AM-treated rabbits. Immunoperoxidase stains showed that the neurofibrillary tangles represented abnormal filamentous accumulations in the perikaryal cytoplasm, immunoreactive with a monoclonal antibody to the 200-kDa subunit of the neurofilament triplet polypeptide; they were nonreactive with monoclonal antibodies to microtubule associated protein 2 (MAP2), tau and the neuron-associated class III ß-tubulin isotype. In the other 10 rabbits in the AM-treated group the OMN was not located. The latter was attributed to the fact that the oculomotor nucleus is a mid-line structure and was "lost" when the cranium was bisected as part of our "rapid" technique to remove the brain from rabbits at necropsy for biochemical as well as morphological study. No lesions were present in the OMN of any of the 17 rabbits in the other two groups in which this nucleus was found.

Direct intraventricular effect of aluminium maltol. We have examined the effects of the direct intraventricular injection of aluminium in New Zealand White rabbits.[34] After the surgical placement of an intraventricular catheter, 100 µl of 25 mmol/L aluminium maltol (3 rabbits) or 75 mmol/L maltol (2 rabbits) was injected postoperatively at timed daily intervals (days 1, 3, 4, 6 and 7). Two animals, which were not treated, were used as controls. The 5 rabbits which received the intraventricular instillation of aluminium maltol developed a widespread neurofibrillary degeneration involving pyramidal neurons of the neocortex and allocortex, projection neurons of the diencephalon, and diverse neuronal populations of the brainstem and spinal cord including the oculomotor nucleus. There was a predilection for motoneuron involvement and for an increased severity of neuronal degeneration in the infratentorial portions of the neuraxis. Perikarya and proximal neurites were especially affected, in contrast to more distal fiber projections. Affected neurons demonstrated intense filamentous immunostaining with a panel of monoclonal antibodies against phosphorylated (SMI-31; Tp-NFP1A3), non-phosphorylated/phosphatase sensitive (SM1-32), and dephosphorylation-independent (SMI-33) epitopes in the high and middle molecular weight neurofilament protein subunits (NF-H/M). By contrast, these lesions were non-reactive with monoclonal antibodies to MAP2, tau, and the class III neuron-associated ß-tubulin isotype. These findings indicate that intraventricular Al maltol produces similar, but more widespread degeneration of projection-type neurons than the less water-soluble Al compounds as previously reported by other workers.

In-vitro Studies

Tissue Culture Studies. We have developed an *in-vitro* neuronal tissue culture system to evaluate the neurotoxic effects of aluminium maltol on foetal rabbit midbrain tissue, containing the oculomotor nucleus.[35] Midbrain explants from 24-day old foetuses were maintained in DMEM-F10 medium with 10% rabbit serum. Cultures were allowed to establish *in vitro* before treatment was commenced. Al-exposed cultures were treated with a final concentration of either 11, 13 or 15 µmol/L Al maltol, while maltol-treated cultures received a final concentration of 39 or 45 µmol/L maltol (molar equivalent to 13 and 15 µmol/L Al maltol). Treated cultures received Al maltol or maltol for 24 or 25 days, while control cultures were maintained on nutrient medium alone for the same period of time.

Argyrophilic neuritic swellings and perikaryal inclusions were produced at 11, 13 and 15 µmol/L Al maltol as compared with maltol and control cultures where the perikaryal inclusions were absent and neuritic swellings were inconspicuous or absent. Perikaryal inclusions were generally, but not always, observed in large neurons and involved only a minority of neurons. Treated cultures, carried for an additional 10 days without any further addition of Al maltol, retained their neuronal perikaryal inclusions and neuritic pathology.

By immunohistochemistry, neuritic swellings and occasional perikarya exhibited reactivity similar to that found in NFTs in our *in-vivo* studies. By electron microscopy, focal accumulations of 10 nm filaments were observed in occasional neuronal somata and neurites of Al-treated explants. Aggregates of intermediate filaments were not seen in the maltol-treated or untreated cultures.

3 CONCLUSION

Because of its ubiquitous presence in the environment, exposure to aluminium cannot be avoided. The mobilization of aluminium from soil and rock by acid rain and its lethal effects on flora and fauna are relevant to its potential for toxic effects on the human species. In patients with impaired renal function, the accumulation of aluminium in tissues is associated with the development of clinical toxic phenomena. Aluminium has been proposed as an etiological factor in a variety of neurological disorders including amyotrophic lateral sclerosis, a form of parkinsonian dementia, Alzheimer's disease and motoneuron disease. Our experimental studies provide evidence that the exposure of brain tissues to aluminium *in vivo* and *in vitro* is associated with a disturbance in the metabolism of cytoskeletal proteins. The use of these experimental systems offers an opportunity to evaluate the potential role of aluminium in the etiology of some neurological disorders.

4 ACKNOWLEDGMENT

Supported by Grant ES04464 of the National Institute of Environmental Health; and by Grant 90-04 from the Commonwealth of Virginia Alzheimer's and Related Diseases Research Award Fund.

5 REFERENCES

1. J. A. T. Pennington, Food Additives and Contaminants, 1987, 5, 161.
2. W. C. Shortle and K. T. Smith, Science, 1988, 240, 1017.
3. C. S. Cronan and C. L. Schofield. Science, 1979, 204, 304.
4. D. W. Schindler, Science, 1988, 239, 149.
5. J. P. Baker and C. L. Schoenfield, Water, Air, Soil Pollution, 1982, 18, 298.
6. C. P. McCahon and D. Pascoe, Arch. Environ. Contam. Toxicol., 1989, 18, 233.
7. R. B. Martin, Clin. Chem., 1986, 32, 1797.
8. G. D. Howells and A. S. Kallend, Chemistry in Britain, 1984, 20, 407.
9. O. K. Skogheim abd B. O. Rosseland, Bull. Environ. Contam. Toxicol., 1986, 37, 258.
10. J. D. Birchall, C. Exley, J. S. Chappell and M. J. Phillips, Nature, 1989, 338, 146.
11. M. R. Wills and J. Savory, CRC Crit. Rev. Clin. Lab. Sci., 1989, 27, 59.
12. A. C. Alfrey, New Engl. J. Med., 1984, 310, 1113.
13. M. M. Platts, G. C. Goode and J. S. Hislop. Brit. Med. J., 1977, 2, 657.
14. D. P. Perl, D. C. Gajdusek, R. M. Garruto, R. T. Yanagihara and C. J. Gibbs, Jr, Science, 1982, 217, 1053.
15. R. J. Wurtman, Scientific American, 1985, 252, 62.
16. R. Katzman, New Engl. J. Med., 1986, 314, 964.
17. J. A. Kwentus, R. Hart, N. Lingon, J. Taylor and J. J. Silverman, Am. J. Med., 1986, 81, 91.
18. I. J. Deary and L. J. Whalley, Brit. Med. J., 1988, 297, 807.
19. C. N. Martyn, C. Osmond, J. A. Edwardson, C. J. P. Barker, E. C. Harris and R. F. Lacey, Lancet, 1989, i, 59.
20. B. Lindegard, Lancet, 1989, i, 267.

21. D. E. Lilienfeld, J. Ehland, P. J. Landrigan, E. Chan, J. Godbold, G. Marsh and D. P. Perl, Lancet, 1989, i, 710.
22. N. H. Sternberger, L. A. Sternberger and J. Ulrich, Proc. Natl. Acad. Sci. USA, 1985, 82, 4274.
23. L. C. Cork, N. H. Sternberger, L. A. Sternberger, M. F. Casanova, R. G. Struble and D. L. Price, J. Neuropathol. Exp. Neurol., 1986, 45, 56. 24. V. M-Y. Lee, L. Otros, Jr., M. L. Schmidt and J. Q. Trojanowski, Proc. Natl. Acad. Sci. USA, 1988, 85, 7384.
25. P. Mulvihill and G. Perry. Brain Res., 1989, 484, 150.
26. L. S. Forno, L. A. Sternberger, N. H. Sternberger, A. M. Strefling, K. Swanson and L. F. Eng, Neurosci. Lett., 1986, 64, 253.
27. M. L. Schmidt, M. J. Carden, V. M-Y. Lee and J. Q. Trojanowski, Lab. Invest., 1987, 56, 282.
28. V. Manetto, N. H. Sternberger, G. Perry, L. A. Sternberger and P. Gambetti, J. Neuropathol. Exp. Neurol., 1988, 47, 642.
29. D. G. Munoz, C. Greene, D. P. Perl and D. J. Selkoe, J. Neuropathol. Exp. Neurol., 1988, 47, 9.
30. H. M. Wisniewski, J. W. Shek, S. Gruca and J. A. Sturman, Acta Neuropathol., 1984, 63, 190.
31. S-H. Yen, D. W. Dickson, C. Peterson and J. E. Goldman, `Progress in Neuropathology,' H. M. Zimmerman (ed), Raven Press, New York, 1986, Vol. 6, p. 72.
32. R. M. Garruto, S. K. Shankar, R. Yanagihara, A. M. Salazar, H. L. Amyx and D. C. Gajdusek, Acta Neuropathol., 1989, 78, 210.
33. R. L. Bertholf, M. M. Herman, J. Savory, R. M. Carpenter, B. C. Sturgill, C. D. Katsetos, S. R. VandenBerg and M. R. Wills, Toxicol. Appl. Pharmacol., 1989, 98, 58.
34. C. D. Katsetos, J. Savory, M. M. Herman, R. M. Carpenter, A. Frankfurter, C. D. Hewitt, and M. R. Wills, Neuropathol. Appl. Neurobiol., 1990, in press.
35. C. D. Hewitt, M. M. Herman, J. Savory and M. R. Wills, International Symposium on Trace Elements in Health and Disease, June 1990, Espoo, Finland (Abstract).

Subject Index

Accuracy, 39
Ageing, 206
Aluminium
  analysis, 3
  neurotoxicity, 219, 227
  release from
    saucepans, 57
Aluminium maltol, 219, 227
  neurotoxicity, 202, 210
Analytical methods, 3
Antioxidants, 201
  antioxidant enzymes, 191
  antioxidant vitamins, 191
Arsenic
  in blood, 88
  in cord blood, 88
  in placenta, 88
Atomic absorption
  spectrometry, 4
Atomic fluorescence
  spectrometry, 29
Beta-carotene, 191
  in heart disease, 132
Biological monitoring, 65
Bismuth chloride, 105
Bismuth subcitrate, 105
Cadmium
  in blood, 75, 95
    smoking effect, 75
    reference levels, 75
  body burden, 95
  in kidney, 95
  in liver, 95
  nephrotoxicity, 95, 209
  in teeth, 69
  toxicokinetics, 95
  in urine, 95
Cancer in experimental animals
  chromium, 165
  nickel, 161
Cancer in humans
  chromium, 163
  nickel, 159
  and selenium, 141
Cardiovascular disease
  trace elements, 127
  vitamins, 127

Catalase, 191
Cell culture, 179, 209
Cell death, 201
Chromium
  carcinogenicity, 163
  in heart disease, 127
Contamination, 13
Copper
  in heart disease, 131
  reference values, 89
EDS analysis, 10, 179
Electron energy loss
  spectroscopy, 11
Electron microscopy, 179, 219
Energy-dispersive
  x-ray analysis, 10, 179
Fetax assay, 169
Free radicals, 191, 201
Genetic predisposition, 71
Glutathione peroxidases, 191
Glutathione transferases, 191
Grid technique, 219
Hydride generation
  techniques, 6
Immunohistochemistry, 219, 227
In vivo perfusion, 105
Individual
  susceptibility, 71
Inductively coupled
  plasma, 7, 8, 19
Isotope separation, 26
Laboratory robotics, 9
Laser fluorescence, 7
Laser microprobe
  mass analysis, 11
Lead
  in blood, 75
    reference levels, 75
    time trends, 75
  in foetal tissues, 109
  intestinal absorption, 109
  secretion in milk, 109
  in teeth, 69
  toxicokinetics, 109
Lipid peroxidation, 191, 201
  in ageing, 206
  and carcinogenesis, 205

Mass spectrometry, 7,8
Matrix modification, 4
Mercury
  analysis, 29
  in blood, 75, 86
  in cord blood, 86
    reference levels, 75
  in hair, 86
  intestinal absorption, 117
  milk transfer, 117
  in placenta, 86
Mesangial renal cells, 209
Methyl mercury
  in blood, 86
  in cord blood, 86
  in hair, 86
  intestinal absorption, 117
  milk transfer, 117
  in placenta, 86
Milk transfer
  lead, 109
  mercury, 117
  methyl mercury, 117
Multielement analysis, 6
Nephrotoxicity
  mechanisms, 209
Neurofilaments, 219, 227
Nickel
  teratogenicity, 169
Nickel subsulfide
  cell transformation, 179
  uptake in cells, 179
Organ culture, 219
Oxide suppression, 18
PCA, 18
Perikaryal tangles, 219, 227
Principal components
  analysis, 18

Proteoglycan synthesis, 212
Quality assessement, 37
Quality assurance, 37
Quality control, 37
Reduced oxygen species, 191
Reference materials, 41
Reference values, 67
  cadmium in blood, 75
  lead in blood, 75
  mercury in blood, 75
  selenium in blood, 75
Reserve capacity, 69
Sample preparation, 13
Selenium
  analysis, 49
  blood levels, 75
    reference values, 75
  role in heart disease, 129
  role in human cancer, 141
  in toe nail clippings, 141
  levels in waters, 53
Specimen collection, 12
Spectral interferences, 20
Superoxide dismutases, 191
Teratogenicity testing
  in frogs, 169
Toxicokinetics, 65
  cadmium, 94
  lead, 109
  mercury, 117
Vitamin C, 191
  in heart disease, 134
Vitamin E, 191
  in heart disease, 133
Xenopus laevis, 169
Zinc
  in heart disease, 130
  reference values, 89